P

"Kicka$$ Happyness"

"If you are lost and have no idea where to begin, this book that is mostly a manual to happiness, will guide you to have the strength to restart your life. If you don't believe in anything else, at least make this your last stop. Try and read it with an open mind because this will shake you and wake you up. Anne Hayes states it very simple and how it is."

Maria F. La Riva
#1 International Bestseller Author
Creator of CreatingYourRealityByMaria.com

"There is personal development...and then there is DEEP Personal Growth. Anne achieves the latter with not only this book, but with the example she sets forth in her own life...this is a must read!"

Steve Hopper
Speaker, Author, and Peak Performance Strategist

"POWERFUL, IMPACTFUL, LIFE-CHANGING!! Anne Hayes shares simple, yet highly effective tools and strategies for 'turbo-charging' and heightening your happiness vibration NOW. The results are IMMEDIATE!
Warning: This book is only for those who are wishing to soar to new heights!"

Susan Hayes (AKA Athena SOL)
The Empowerment Extraordinaire
Speaker, Author, Mentor

"Empowering, Authentic, and Motivating! Anne, aka Mama G, will give you such a level of awareness, that by the time you are done reading this book, you will not have only found an amazing amount of true 'Happyness', but also an increased sense of accomplishment! Everyone who reads this book will be on fire!"

Jose Flores
Global Mindset Disruptor, Motivational Speaker, and Author of <u>Don't Let Your Struggle Become Your Standard</u>

"As I read the pages of the book, I could hear the author's joy exude through the page as it was leading me through a defined path to happiness. There were so many authentic and practical truths shared in this book that makes happiness feel like an innocent kid enjoying ice cream on a hot summer day. Although Anne acknowledges that happiness takes intentional work, reading this book made it seem like I had a happiness coach walking me through every step of the way. Great read!"

Dr. Ursula T. Wright
Founder of Color the World Labs and Faithruption United

"As someone who reads a lot of personal development books, I wasn't expecting to be so impacted by this one — but I was! Anne has a fresh, infectious, high-vibe style that is so easy and fun to read, while at the same time going deep with wisdom for living a fulfilling life. Anne's no-BS approach to healing and stepping into "happyness" is just what I needed (and didn't know it). I highly recommend this book if you're looking for a hefty dose of inspiration and conscious motivation."

Michelle Villalobos
CEO & Founder, Superstar Activator

Kicka$$ Happyness

HOW TO STEP INTO YOUR AUTHENTIC POWER WITH GRACE AND CREATE THE LIFE YOU DESIRE

Brought into this Reality Upon Your Request

ANNE HAYES (AKA MAMA G)
THE EMPOWERMENT QUEEN

Collective Creator of Kicka$$ Happyness

AH
ANNE HAYES
Self-published

Library of Congress Cataloging-in-Publication Data has been applied for.

ISBN: 978-1-7344728-0-6

I'd like to dedicate this book to all the healers on my journey who understood on a deeply spiritual level, what I truly needed to move forward in my life.

Their innate gifts, unconditional love, and devoted compassion were all critical components in my ability to activate higher states of consciousness and awareness

. They guided me in transforming my past pain into fuel for a fantastically fabulous future by becoming more powerfully present in ongoing "NOW" moments. T

They were instrumental in bringing me to my "Happy Space". ☺

True Happiness... is not attained through self-gratification,
but through fidelity to a worthy purpose.
-Helen Keller

TABLE OF (BEYOND) CONTENT!

ACKNOWLEDGEMENTS

Where to begin? It is a challenge to reach back and truly understand the grand scope of the experiences that led up to the creation of this book, from a truly "HAPPY" place.

I choose to begin with my inception into this reality, birthed by a mother full of love and compassion and a commitment to family values. To add to this unconditional maternal sweetness was a dad who instilled in me a sense of adventure and excitement through creative resourcefulness. Together, my parents taught me to boldly and playfully navigate this Earthly playground.

Of course, I'd be remiss if I didn't mention my 5 siblings, including my twin sister, who, along with our extended family and a multitude of friends and acquaintances, filled my days with love, support, encouragement, and a sense of belonging...

and sometimes, an opportunity to grow, to learn, and to evolve through unexpected challenges.

You see, having the level of awareness and the knowledge and understanding that I now possess, I can't help but be incredibly grateful for the role that each of us chose to take on in this "Earth School" Environment. And so, where once there was judgement, frustration, sadness, even anger and rage, there is now a sense of peace that has the ability to unfold into what I call "Kicka$$ Happyness".

And so I acknowledge being both the perpetrator and the victim, the judge and the judged, the lover and the hater, the aggressor and the suppressor, the secret and the truth, the brave and the weak, the darkness and the light, and everything in between.

ACKNOWLEDGEMENTS

With this, I offer my gratitude for every single person, circumstance, situation, event, and experience that has landed on my journey, the perceived good, bad and the ugly; for it has catapulted me in a way I never thought possible, until NOW! :)

With Sincerest Appreciation,

Anne Hayes/Mama G

FOREWORD

Great wondrous day reader. We are a unique stream of consciousness from the Angelic Realm that has chosen to engage with you in more ways than you could possibly yet conceive.

We have chosen to become a part of your experience as another critical component in raising the vibration of the planet.

You see, we have witnessed a marked and dangerous increase in mental illness with an overwhelming occurrence of especially anxiety-related disorders and deep depression. We have also seen the reports from the CDC regarding the leap in suicide deaths in the last decade among now your pre-teen population in the U.S.

And so it is with great honor that we welcome you to an experience as a reader that will not only undoubtedly uplift YOU, but those around you as well. In fact, we anticipate a reverberatory effect beyond time and space that links us all back to the Divine and its Grace.

Anne is living proof that one can overcome the most seemingly severe forms of trauma and associated mental illness. OCD, debilitating anxiety, panic attacks, deep despair, raging anger, sinking shame, unhealthy compliance, low self-esteem, false confidence, and a fatalistic view on life can ALL be transformed to extreme confidence, peace of mind, inner peace, gentle acceptance, compelling compassion, magical manifestation, and a KICKA$$ HAPPY ELEVATED VIBRATION"!

FOREWORD

And so use this book as a method to refocus your efforts and your awareness in a way that aligns with Universal Principles set in motion by a Most Supreme, Benevolent Infinite Creator.

You DESERVE to be Happy! It is your Birthright!

-The Angelic Realm

INTRODUCTION

"Happiness is when what you think, what you say, and what you do are in harmony." **-Mahatma Ghandi**

"Happiness of your life depends on the quality of your thoughts." **-Marcus Aurelius**

"Happiness understands, accepts and celebrates that absolutely everything happens FOR you as an ongoing gift from a Divine Source." **-Mama G**

I'm not here to say that I will empower you to step into your Authentic Power with High-soaring Happiness, in an instant, although instantaneous combustion is possible. It can happen in this way, if you've already done most of the legwork yourself, and are ready to sprout, so to speak!

More likely, your Extreme, Unshakeable, Unbreakable Confidence to do just that will show itself when all the conditions are just right (ripe), conditions that You, Yourself, have put into place and activated! And I truly believe that this book may be the critical catalyst you have been looking for to finally acquiesce what you desire!

And so I have shown up in your experience, just as you have called, to simply give you a **turbocharge** on both your personal and professional growth, almost like a jumpstart. From there, you will provide the fuel for accelerated growth through your ongoing, committed action steps towards what success looks like for you, with a bit of cruise control that you establish along the way.

INTRODUCTION

Think of me like a compass that helps to set you in the right direction for your life, a North Star that guides you to all your deepest desires, so long as you remain focused and are willing to consistently implement the strategies shared in this book.

Furthermore, the insights and perspectives found in this book will come alive as you openly receive them into your updated operating system of beliefs, infusing you with a new elevated energy signature.

However, please understand that there is nothing to overcome. You are already there, or shall I say, here. ☺ It's simply a matter of you finding the keys to unlock your own innate gifts that await your courage to access them through the doors of unlimited possibilities, so that you can experience what it is to feel truly **Happy**!

What you will require:

1. Commitment to take action
2. A strong desire to change NOW
3. A deep willingness to let go of any preconceived notions about what <u>Authentic Power</u> looks like
4. A Genuine Intention to Focus on Your Own **Happiness**!
5. Gratitude
6. Patience

X_____

Sign here to honor your commitment to yourself!

Grab your jetpacks, and hold onto your hats!
It's time to Take Off!!!!

CHAPTER 1

Honor Yourself
Allow Yourself Time to Heal

"Healing is an art.
It takes time.
It takes practice.
It takes love."
-Anonymous

"Setting time aside to take care of yourself is not being selfish. It is honoring yourself."
-Nyambura Mwangi

"Taking the time to heal ourselves is the highest form of self-love. It allows us to show up in the World, standing in our most <u>Authentic Power</u>."
-Mama G

Whew! What a whirlwind it has been! I'm guessing that life has "kicked you in the pants" multiple times, and that you may be feeling a bit exhausted at this point. Because, somehow, on some level, you experienced a traumatic period or event that left you feeling like you've been "bullied" on the playground of life. You've cried out, have lost your way, perhaps your faith, and even your will to live.

You might have said to yourself, "Is this as good as it gets? Really? I don't remember signing up for this! What's the dang purpose of all this?"

In fact, you might have said on more than a few occasions (like I did)...

LIFE SUCKS!

Well, the great news, is that if you've picked up this book, you are already beyond this deep level of negativity. You want more, and you know there is more. You simply want to feel better, right NOW!

Well, guess what? You came to the right place. Feel better yet?

Great! Let's remove this perspective right NOW!

~~LIFE SUCKS!~~

Let's speak life into this, instead:

"Life is not happening to me; it is happening FOR me, always."

(Say aloud every day as reminder!)

Now let me continue by "validating" your experience, your pain, your perspective, and anything else that has created your present challenge. Having been where you are, I "get it"; it takes time to remove the layers of protection we have wrapped ourselves in, an adaptation for survival in a World that has often seemed reckless and uncaring.

Let me share that at one time, I too, was not yet ready to take ownership of the life that I had created; built on all too familiar past experiences and my constant state of worry about creating more of the same. You see, my lack of awareness and an outdated system of beliefs allowed the demons of self-doubt to creep into my mind, my body, AND my spirit in a way that was detrimental to my overall well-being!

You see, I often felt like a victim and sought to blame everybody and everything, but myself. I looked for excuse after excuse for settling for a more or less ho hum life. In fact, my victim mentality created more circumstances that had me feeling like a victim. My closest relationships became strained, I was all too judgmental of both others and myself, I developed a very negative attitude, I became very easily frustrated, and eventually became very depressed and physically ill at my seeming inability to change the course of my life. My state of mind for a long time, said, "Stop the World, I want to get off."

In fact, it was this state of mind that created my state of being. And this state of being, in turn, appeared to nibble away at my happiness like the incessant tapping of a woodpecker on a weathered home. It seemed to leave gaping holes in my soul that begged for repair.

So basically, I GET it!

And so, how does one begin to get that Extreme, KICKA$$ HAPPYNESS back, the HAPPYNESS with the Confidence that says I am bodacious, courageous, ready to turn the pages, be the sage, and just, take back **my <u>POWER!</u>**

And so where to begin? Well, for starters, it helps to start with "starters"! ☺ This is like an appetizer that prepares us for the Grand Meal that includes dessert and coffee and then some, if we choose, as we create the "next grandest version of the greatest vision we ever had of ourselves." (I'd like to own that one, but that one belongs to Neale Donald Walsch, author of the <u>Conversations with God</u> series).

So let's get "started"....by simply NOT starting. "Wait. What? NOT starting? What in the World does that mean?" you ask.

It means just that, like setting the table, and placing a napkin on your lap before you eat. It means take a break, take your time, express some gracious gratitude for what lays in front of you, and then begin slowly with a few nibbles on that protective layering that has created a barrier between you and the life you have envisioned for yourself.

"Why so?" as you question my sanity. Because a lifetime of events fueled by self-defeating thoughts cannot be gobbled up in just one sitting. Truth be told, it can actually make you very, very sick, and leave you immobile once again, moaning and groaning and grasping at your belly. That's not what we want here.

What we seek, instead, is to offer you a gentle remembrance of WHO YOU REALLY ARE. And WHO YOU REALLY ARE is a KICKA$$ Superstar ready to
"Activate Your Authenticity" (I don't own that one either! That belongs to my sister, Susan Hayes, of Solactiviation.com), but collective minds ought to share!

And so begin with your healing. You do NOT have to identify your purpose in life, have crystal clear vision, and a stack of money in your bank account to bring yourself into the ever present moment where life really happens!

Instead, find a way to step back from your responsibilities so that you can design a day with limited routines and ample time for rest, self-reflection, and an opportunity to breathe deeply.

Now, this may take some creative problem-solving on your part, but it absolutely CAN and SHOULD be done if you truly want to develop the type of Authentic Power that is going to help you to grow and expand into the joyfully abundant life that I know you desire.

Healing=Transformation=Increased Power and Authenticity
=Kicka$$ Happyness

EQUALS...

I am ready to get out there and do whatever it takes to create the life I envision for myself!

And so, what exactly might it look like to step back?

It might involve moving into a smaller home, moving in with a family member or friend, working from home more often, asking for help more often, soliciting the help of your children, if you have children, with household chores, including the preparation of dinner, carpooling, or cutting back on unnecessary expenses. It might even include sleeping on a mattress in your living room while renting out your room or collecting cans and scrapping metal.

Guess what? I pretty much did ALL of the above! Although I was fortunate enough to collect a monthly security check for my two children after I became a widow early on in their lives, it wasn't nearly enough to support the lifestyle we had created; not unless I chose to work full-time, and struggle to pay for child care while I dealt with the overwhelming task of healing myself. I opted for my healing and for the healing of my family.

This was not an easy choice, especially as our family seemed to endure more financial struggles than those around us. I also felt I had to say, "no", to my children more often than I would have liked. Furthermore, it appeared as though others were jealous of the fact that I could choose to work only part-time or not at all. However, I don't believe my family and friends could have ever come to understand the scope of my pain and my struggle.

And so, I say, honor yourself. Practice self-care. Read more often. Soak up the sun. Take more walks. Talk warm baths. Sip your coffee, your tea, or your water. Take up yoga. Plant a garden. Hug a tree. Listen to soothing music. Sleep in. Book a massage if you're able. Breathe more deeply. Admire more sunsets. Swim in the ocean. Journal.

Take time to Heal.   Take time to Heal.

Take time to Heal.

Think of this as "Your Reconstruction Phase", a complete renovation to include marbled floors, balconies with majestic views, and stainless steel appliances, all with a backsplash of increasing **happiness** and peace of mind. In fact, you can envision what that would look like for you, right NOW!

1.   What does it feel like to be **Happier** than you've ever felt in your life?
2.   How do you stand, walk, interact with others?
3.   How do others talk and respond to you?
4.   How does it feel in your body?
5.   What emotions do you experience?
6.   Look around. Where are you spending most of your time? Describe your environment.
7.   What kind of friends are you now hanging out with?
8.   What do your relationships look like?
9.   How is your **"happiness"** now showing up?
10.   What scents/aromas come into your awareness?
11.   How does it physically feel to be a person who experiences a generally truly **happy** demeanor?
12.   What does the **Happier** You look like to others, to you?
13.   In what kind of activities are you now engaged? What choices do you make?
14.   What does it feel like to be excited about life?

"Whoa, wait a minute," some of you might say..."I don't need this list, and I don't need any healing! My life is good. I just want to feel a little more **happy**, more of the time! I'm as 'real' as they get! A self-renovation??? That's not me!"

Well, that's what I thought. You see, I had been on a journey for years, healing myself and successfully helping others to heal as well. I was contributing in a lot of ways. However, despite all my new skills and the increased investment in myself on many levels, I was still lacking the high level type of Kicka$$ Vibrational Frequency that would allow me to *attract* the lifestyle I had been dreaming of. Without realizing it, I was still attached to what others thought of me. I backed away from true **Power** by building my success on the positive praise of others. Furthermore, I was under the illusion that I could get everyone to like me. As a lesbian living in the Bible Belt here in the U.S., I wasn't yet ready to take on what I call the "self-haters" that believed that I was someone to be tolerated and not necessarily celebrated.

In fact, I became disheartened that despite all my efforts and the time and the money I had invested in myself and in my business, I still wasn't making the progress I had hoped. Now there were clearly other factors that showed up that "appeared" on the surface to impede my growth. However, it also became crystal-clear to me at one point, that to some, it just didn't matter how inspirational or loving I was. It didn't matter how much experience I had. It didn't matter how much value I could bring to others. I was a lesbian, and I didn't belong. I didn't fit into the belief systems of the community in which I found myself. Now, intellectually, I knew it wasn't personal. But dang, did it take some time and some pain to move from the intellectual to the experiential understanding of this.

And so for a while, I seemed to sputter and flail as I swam in unchartered, "troubling for me" waters. I connected with as many people as I could. I was honest about who I WAS, and AM. I shared my story. But after two years of climbing uphill in my mind, I felt I needed a desperate respite. There seemed to be too many "opened, and then closed" doors, and I kept being passed up.

I jumped back into the trench, sitting on the bench, with a gut wrench in my belly, because I KNEW that it truly came down....

Came down...

Came all the way

D

O

W

N...

to my *"fear of rejection"*.

And that's what allowed the self-sabotaging self-doubt to continue to work its way back into my thoughts, like a serpent furtively making its way through the tall grass of emotional triggers attached to past events. I was all too often "trigger happy", but not necessarily happy about the way my life seemed to be unfolding at the time.

And so for me, it required even MORE healing! And I didn't do it alone. I leaned on others, sought insight, amped up my skill set, and continued to learn, to develop, and to consistently implement powerful practices that I will share with you in this book.

Why am I taking the time to do this?

Because I genuinely want you, and anyone else who picks up this book, to walk away with a sense of accomplishment for taking the next steps to instilling within yourself the most "Hip to the Heightened Happy Vibe", so that you can step into your most Authentic Power to Create, Create, Create a Most Cherished Life!

And so here's to the next level of your transformation!

I'm excited to be sharing this journey with you!

Major Action Step:

Come up with at least one thing you can do this week to begin to lighten your "load", so that you can allow more time for personal healing and transformation.

CHAPTER 2

Practice Deep Self-reflection
Tap into the Source of Infinite Knowledge

*"Don't become too preoccupied with what is happening around you.
Pay more attention to what is going on within you."*
-Mary-Frances Winters

"Stars are holes in the sky from which the Infinite shines."
-Confucius

"Go within with the help of a calming, soothing breath to unveil the gift of awareness."
-Mama G

Fantastic! Now that you have created more down time for yourself, let's utilize it in the best manner possible! Now, it's ok to watch a little Netflix or watch a little TV, but if you're looking to turbocharge your expansion, then I suggest you limit this particular activity!

Now, so you know, I don't ever subscribe to the grind, grind, grind 10x mentality. I believe it goes against our nature, and can create an unhealthy balance in our lives that can bring

about adversity on many levels. To me, this is an egoic approach to success, sometimes planted too deeply in a 3D construct where our dreams may never take root.
I liken it to planting seeds too deeply with a bit too much vigor. This obsessive approach which I believe is somewhat fear-based (I have to overperform, overproduce to flourish the way that I desire.) plants an exorbitant amount of seeds with often exhaustive energetic output with the hope that the moisture and the warmth will somehow reach the depths of one's excessive efforts.

Now, this can and often does produce results, as Grant Cardone of the 10X philosophy has proven time and time again.

Yet, *what if, what if*...the same results could be produced with more ease, using your innate, Divine skills more efficiently, as a way to collapse time and space, so that you didn't have to encounter years of pushing through painful memories to attain the type of **Kicka$$ Happyness** (as a precursor to the financial wealth and personal success) that many wish for?

What if you were able to schedule in more time for your loved ones, your friends, and most importantly, yourself?

What if the healing process could be simplified and expedited like Amazon on demand, 24/7, when you needed it the most?

What if you took the words ~~sacrifice~~, ~~paying the price~~, ~~working long hours~~, and ~~waiting years and years~~ to sow what you could reap? What if there were more highly advanced methods and readily available tools that you could use, RIGHT NOW, that would most surely allow you to better enjoy the journey? Would you want that? Would you be willing to minimize the short term losses for more sustainable, even more extraordinary long-term gains?

My guess is that your answer to all of these is a resounding, "Yes! Heaven on Earth, Yeah!"

Well, then let's dig in...but not too deep (ha ha), unless it's a deeply meditative *alpha or **theta state.

Now, let's leave the marijuana alone here, if possible, because it is absolutely possible to attain these states all on your own. However, it will take practice and perhaps some perseverance, at first, to develop the habit of easily checking in with your own intuition, your own gut instinct, your own Divine Guidance, your Higher Self, God, Source, the Quantum Field....whatever you want to call "It". If you believe it, and you have faith, it will work!

*An **alpha state** of mind" is lower frequency brain wave activity just below an actively awake "beta state of mind" where creativity, imagination, and intuition are more easily accessed (https://www.wikihow.com)

A "theta state** of mind" is a deep meditative state that allows for an even greater flow of creative ideas and the ability to self-program in a dream-like state. The theta state exists at a lower frequency than the alpha state. Mental relaxation through gentle respiration allows us to access these states. (https://www.wikihow.com)

Ok, so HOW does it actually work? Well, let's begin by reviewing the body's response to stress as opposed to the body's response to the breath.

In doing so, however, it is important to note that there is in fact, a very clear connection between the body, the mind, and the spirit. A change in one will undoubtedly effect a change in the other two.

Let's begin with stress. Stress, according to my good old friend, Google, is *"a state of mental or emotional strain or tension resulting from adverse or very demanding circumstances"*. Working too hard (the "grind" mentality), fatigue from lack of sleep or worry, an unfavorable pattern of thinking, or reliving a traumatic event are each enough to trigger the sympathetic nervous system* into action. The perceived threat to the body triggers a signal to be sent to the body which responds by releasing hormones known as adrenaline and cortisol. Together, these hormones help to regulate particular functions in the body, so that the body is prepared to "fight or take flight". This emergency response causes an increase in one's heart rate, increased blood flow to the extremities and away from vital organs (for quick, fast movement if needed), an increase in blood sugar for a quick burst of energy, more rapid breathing, tense muscles, and beads of sweat on the skin.

*Sympathetic nervous system: A part of the **nervous system** that serves to accelerate the heart rate, constrict blood vessels, and raise blood pressure. (https://www.wikihow.com)

Now, if you think about it, it's incredible that the body does this automatically. We do not have to command our body to respond in any of these ways. In fact, it is designed to keep us safe, to protect us, and to help us to survive any threat to our overall well-being. This is an absolutely wonderful function that clearly has practical use in our lives. For example, it's great to know that we are instantly pulled into heightened awareness with laser sharp focus and the ability to move quickly AND with agility when a speeding car sharply rounds the corner as we are about to cross the street or when a wildly agitated animal crosses our path. It is often the difference between life and death.

However, however...back to the "stress" part. Now, let me stress (I couldn't help it.) that short-lived stress in response to a viable threat is actually healthy for the reasons I stated above. However, and this is where it becomes a bit "loopy", literally! When we receive ongoing threats (such as repeated trauma), we develop a neural network in our brains that actually triggers a repeated, energy-depleting response to any situation remotely familiar to the initial ongoing threat.

We keep "looping" back, expressing a similar pattern of thinking, behaving, acting AND reacting until we are able to heal. For example, someone who has ever been shot, is likely to react instinctively anytime there is a loud noise, such as a car backfiring or fire crackers being lit up. As you might imagine, this ongoing heightened reaction is likely to place the body in a state of chronic stress. I liken it to a "Trap" beat with a repetitive, almost hypnotic play on our senses of hearing and touch (pulsating beat) along with a disruption to our electromagnetic field due to the often discordant frequency of the beat.

Now so you know, I am an emcee. I write inspirational rap and hip hop, and I highly value the gift of these musical genres, including "Trap"* as a form of expression. However, I also understand the effect that certain frequencies of music can have on our bodily systems and rhythms.

The lyrics are also critical as they help to speak life into that which we want to show up in our lives. The idea that "sticks and stones can break my bones, but words can never hurt me" is ignorant to the power of both unspoken and spoken words. In fact, it has been scientifically proven that both thoughts and words carry energy frequencies which affect our reality (this is the field of quantum physics as well as a basic biblical principle!). We'll delve deeper into this in chapter 4.

Until then, let's discuss the importance of creating a new "loop" or pattern of thoughts, much like re-piping a house or reprogramming a computer. This reprogramming is essential to our survival. I know, sounds like a paradox, and in a sense, it is. But to keep the Sympathetic Nervous System from becoming overtaxed, we must become more adept at distinguishing between true threats and those fabricated in our minds. Otherwise, we become physically, mentally, and emotionally exhausted over time, and this can often lead to disease.

*Trap music is a form of Hip Hop that came out of the Southern U.S. in and around 2000 with a typically melancholy, dark ambient "tone" with lyrics to match. (https://www.wikihow.com)

Referring back to the computer analogy, if we were to imagine our brain as the hardware and our mind as that which provides the software through our most dominant thought patterns, then we would simply need to update our operating system to a more advanced, more expansive system of beliefs. This would help to create a more favorable personal reality for us. This is what we call transformation. And to become the super Happy person that shows up with the Gracious **Authentic Power** to Create, then this transformation is a MUST. The other option is to remain unchanged and literally chained to a network that has long become outdated.

So HOW do we go about reprogramming ourselves? Weren't we born with personalities that remain throughout our lifetimes? Doesn't our DNA dictate who we are and how we respond to events in our lives? Is it actually possible to recover from trauma?

All great questions! First of all, we can absolutely fully recover from trauma! Secondly, we can actually change our DNA, and we can in fact, change our personalities! Yes, you read that right! We can in fact, change our personalities! We can even change the very essence of who we are, but that's not something we'd likely wish to do in this particular experience. But yes, the personality we create as our Identity creates our personal reality. It's more commonly known as personal transformation. That's something I learned from the famous, international speaker and neuroscientist, Joe Dispenza, author of <u>Becoming Supernatural: How Common People Are Doing the Uncommon</u>. It is partly due to his groundbreaking work, along with many others, that I am writing this book today!

It's the whole caterpillar in the chrysalis analogy where the caterpillar undergoes an incredible metamorphosis to become a delicate, majestic butterfly. Ah, the teachings of nature. Isn't nature just amazing? I believe so!

Before we get to the "HOW" of metamorphosis, however, let me have you briefly ponder the following:

What if a grumpy, bitter, generally negative person were able to become a pleasant, grateful, typically positive and upbeat person?

Do you believe it would change how life shows up for this person? Do you believe this person would experience more joy, more meaningful relationships, more abundance, more opportunities?

ABSOLUTELY!!

I know because that was me! I did not like to admit it at the time, but I was once a very negative, easily angered and frustrated, depressed person. I had debilitating anxiety, uncontrollable OCD, and spent a lifetime distracting myself from the pain I did not want to feel that stemmed from repeated sexual trauma as a child. Looking back, there were many minor situations that felt like an ominous threat to me, and I reacted in a way that exemplified my struggle.

So, what finally put me on the track to achieve this level of personal transformation? For me, it was an opportunity for long periods of deep reflection, meditation, walks in nature, and yoga. I also listened to soothing music and began to more closely monitor my diet. I became more mindful of what I put into my body and into my mind. I also learned, practiced, and became trained in a number of alternative healing modalities that saw me grow exponentially in a short amount of time.

My gateway to **happiness**, to ultra-transformative healing, however, was yoga. I cried the first time I attended a class, and it was incredibly cathartic. Surprisingly, I was told by the instructor at the time, that this was pretty typical! I guess I had an excessive amount of pain to let go of, because I must have cried for the first 2 years I attended yoga classes. In fact, there was one particularly gifted and inspirational instructor who kept me moving forward when I wasn't sure I had the strength to do so. I admired her fit, tone body, the personable and compassionate way she connected with the participants, and the fact that she seemed to be completely enamored by her chosen path in life. I wanted all of that, and so I kept going back for more.

At the same time that I was attending sometimes 3 yoga classes a week, I sought the help of a local gifted healer who first introduced me to *Reiki. More crying. Lots of crying! This also included me rolling around on my living room floor in fits and spasms of me pounding my fists on the rug and kicking my feet. I also often screamed and sobbed and cried for 45

*Reiki: a healing technique based on the principle that the therapist can channel energy into the patient to activate the natural healing processes of the patient's body and restore physical and emotional well-being (https://www.wikihow.com)

minutes or more. Of course, this usually happened when my kids were in school and I was home alone. As an aside, it made me wonder, since I was living in Salem, MA at the time, if this is what really happened during the Salem Witch Trials. Perhaps Tituba had special healing powers not yet recognized or accepted. Maybe it was the "demons" of pain and fear and the attachment to the ego, that were causing these girls to exhibit such seemingly bizarre behavior. Because honestly, that was me! I was releasing "demons".

Let me emphasize. This reaction occurred almost every time following one of these energy healing sessions. Fortunately they became less severe over time. For me, it was a clear indication that I was healing, that the pain that had lain dormant in me for so long, was finding release. And I was finding a great deal of relief. I was generally **happier**, felt more at peace, became more compassionate, and increased my self-awareness. I grew tremendously.

I grew because all of these activities greatly reduced the destructive nature of my stress by improving the quality of my breath (Anyone ever tell you to just count to 10?).
This in turn helped me to increase my level of awareness about how I was showing up in the World. Furthermore, I was able to clearly receive the intuitive guidance that provided me with both the insight and the action steps that would bring me into greater and greater alignment with WHO I truly WAS and AM. In fact, I believe there is a Source of Infinite Knowledge that we might call God, the Divine, the Quantum Field, or a number of other ways to identify this backing of faith in our lives. And when we choose to listen to this Source, our lives unfold with the greatest of ease and grace, because

this Source/this God/this Divine Being is on call 24/7 and always ready to receive and to grant our greatest desires.

With all that being said, let's return to the power of the breath in its ability to connect us to our subconscious mind and the seat of our soul. When we are able to slow down our breath and to inhale fully and exhale completely, we harmoniously bring together our mind, our body, and our spirit. This clears the pathway to that enlightened aspect of ourselves. It removes mental chatter and the feelings of doubt, allowing for a stronger connection. And connect we must, if we are to reprogram our subconscious mind with the new beliefs we have established about how life can and will show up for us.

And so take the time to "tap in". Do it often. Elevate your mood to one of gratitude. Breathe it in. And then imagine the new and improved you, engaging all of the senses to perceive how that would look for you!

To help get you started, I am going to share a very brief meditation with you on the next page.

(Read it aloud to yourself or have someone else read it to you.)

LETTING GO

Take a few deep breaths. Part of letting go is breathing deeply so that you can move the oxygen around, and give yourself space to release.

Imagine as you breathe, that you can see the breath. It is a combination of sky blue/cobalt blue liquid moving throughout your body with ease. As it moves throughout your body, it picks up what your body doesn't want. Imagine it flowing through your heart and grabbing all the hurt feelings brought about by anything anyone might have said or done that didn't make you feel good. It then flows down below your ribcage into your abdomen. It picks up feelings of sadness and boredom before moving on to your spleen where it picks up feelings you might have ever felt about being left out or feeling as though you didn't belong. From here, this vibrant, cleansing liquid moves up just below your ribs, washing away any fear or anxiety that you might have or have had about anything. From here, the liquid proceeds toward the throat and removes any pain you may have felt when someone used words to hurt you or when you didn't feel as though others wanted to listen to you. Finally, this liquid flows into your head, taking away feelings of confusion and loneliness.

Now, take another deep breath and as you exhale, push out this liquid breath so that it takes away all the unpleasant emotions and feelings with it as it goes.

Then, imagine this liquid becoming heated by a warm sun and evaporating into the air. Feel yourself become lighter, like a balloon ready to float upward. You have now created the space for what your body wants and what YOU want! :)

On the next breath in, visualize yourself breathing in luxurious liquid sunshine (the same sunshine that evaporated what you just breathed out) that gradually fills up your entire body. As you do this, imagine breathing in a sense of belonging, ... confidence, ...happiness,... courage,... love,... understanding,... and peace. Smile as you do so. Continue to breathe easily and effortlessly.

Take at least a few minutes to bask in this renewal.

If you enjoyed this meditation and are interested in more like it, you can go to https://annehayes360.com/ to purchase my book entitled, Teenage Grace/La Gracia del Joven, a book of simple, yet powerful one-page meditations.

You can also visit my SoundCloud @ https://soundcloud.com/kickasshappyness to listen to the MP3 version of each of these meditations for free. ☺

Let me back up a little here. If meditation is not your thing just yet ☺, I suggest you find other quiet activities to soothe your mood. You may have to exercise vigorously, first, so that you can release toxins as well as endorphins! Activity primes you for the right type of elevated mood to gain the most from meditation.

I personally was only able to meditate for very short periods at one time. Highly disturbing images seemed to crash into my mind, and my inability to control them created an extreme aversion to sitting still, let alone meditating. I had what I've already mentioned, debilitating anxiety. I rarely took a full breath (this was before I began practicing yoga), I rushed to fit in a what seemed to be a million activities in one day, ate mindlessly, exercised fanatically, and basically plowed through my existence with my focus on the struggle of my past and the worry about my future. Rarely was I present in the present. The good news is that the development of new, more healthy habits through determined and then gentle, consistent practice, reaped its rewards!

I slowly freed myself from the grip of trauma and victimhood. I began to breathe more freely, to trust more, to feel more safe, and to gravitate to the wisdom of the greatest sages throughout the greatest ages! I became that golden girl drinking that golden milk *(*See Appendix A for the recipe!)*.

Major Action Step:
Choose at least one modality or activity that you can commit to doing at least 10 minutes every day where you are able to calm the breath, so that you can "tap in".

Here are some suggestions:
*Take a walk.
*Listen to soothing and calming music.
*Listen to an Inspirational Video.
*Pray.
*Meditate
*Practice Yoga.
*Sit in nature and breathe in the fresh air.
*Sit for 10 minutes and do NOTHING!

*Lie on your bed and place one hand on your chest and one on your belly as you breathe gently in and out.
*Hug a tree.
*Watch a sunrise or a sunset.

For a list of activities that can help you to heal, to better connect with Source (God), to further your awareness and deepen your intuitive abilities, refer to Appendix B.

CHAPTER 3

Focus on Your Amazing Attributes
Own Your Unique Gifts

"Embrace your uniqueness. You are different, your gift is special - own it and unapologetically share it with the world."
-Oprah Winfrey

"To be yourself in a world that is constantly trying to make you something else is the greatest accomplishment."
-Ralph Waldo Emerson

"There is absolutely no one who can do what you do in the way that you do it! Once you realize this, the idea of competition will fade from your memory, and you will shine with all the other stars to light up the darkest night!"
-Mama G

Congratulations! You are well on the healing journey that is going to transform you with the "greatest, float like a butterfly, Muhammad Ali- like", steadfast confidence,

happily doing what you love most! You are stepping into your Authentic Power and Transforming to the Greatness that is already within you!!! You are now accustomed to deeper self-reflection. And you have developed the uncanny ability to connect with a wealth of limitless knowledge that is always at the tips of your awareness! You are a pioneer ready to blaze a trail with the unique gifts Divinely designed into your Being! So become your amazing self by stepping into and embracing these gifts, today, right NOW! Be that special flower that opens and flourishes in all its glory, right next to all the very different, but equally amazing flowers in what I call, "the garden variety of life"!

If you like to sing, sing your heart out. Share it with the World. Perhaps you like to cook, design costumes, create dance routines, produce music, develop software, play soccer, write poetry, make flower arrangements, engineer new projects, build models, design state of the art homes, solve algebraic equations, code new Alexa skills, garden, share jokes, rescue animals, nurture others, volunteer, photograph picturesque scenes. Whatever it is, do more of it! Develop it. Practice it. Embrace it. Share it!

Why? Because when we take those especially unique skills and talents which are part of our natural make up, and foster them, then it provides a sense of joy and upliftment, not only for us, but for the World!

Here's the key, though. It must be a gift which is not forced into existence because you want to fit in, because it seems to be a trend, or because it's cool to be able to do it. In other words, don't show up for soccer tryouts when you'd rather be at the local skate park, because there appears to be a certain level of prestige in making the soccer team. Vice versa, don't hang out at the skate park with your new Vans just to look cool when you'd rather be playing soccer. You see, to be truly Happy and standing in your <u>Authentic Power</u>, you must be YOU and only YOU, in all its fantastically, fabulously amazing uniqueness. Basically, stay in your lane! Otherwise, you'll be bumping up against those in their full expression, disrupting the smooth flow of grace on the byways of life. Take the high way and be true to you. Be real. Be transparent. Be authentic, because if you're not, you may crash and burn and end up in the break down lane once again. Instead, keep moving forward, stay focused, be patient, be consistent, stay determined, have trust, build faith, and believe in yourself!

This last part is critically important. Although it's great to have others believe in you, if you wait on and depend on this, there will surely be many who DON'T believe in you. Then what? Who do you listen to? Nobody, but YOU and your own instincts! Take a lesson out of *Gary V's playbook, and be your own cheerleader, your own believer, your own achiever, intrinsically motivated because you just love what you're doing!

That's called passion. If you're doing it or talking about it, and your friends don't see your eyes light up, can't feel the animation in your voice, then you may want to check in with

* Gary Vaynerchuk is a Belarusian American entrepreneur, New York Times best-selling author, speaker and Internet personality. (https://www.wikihow.com)

yourself. Fall back on the introspection and the awareness around what you're doing. Then get back to what makes your heart swell, and I'm not talking about romance here, unless you're romancing your gifts!

Fall in love with LIFE!

That's exactly what I began to do after the death of my partner 10 years ago. For me, my high became, and still is, writing lyrics to a variety of Hip Hop beats, and freestyling. I don't do it because I want to connect with the teens I feel destined to serve. I do it because I've been gifted with the ability to do it with so much ease and so much joy. It is effortless for me, and I believe it can be the same for you regarding whatever specific talent or skill rocks your own World!

Now, you might say, this is great, but how do I make money doing what I love to do? That's up to you to figure out. The important thing to understand is that it's been done thousands, perhaps millions of times over and over. It is possible to earn oodles of cash doing what you love while also helping others.

Here are some examples:

Bill Gates is an American business magnate, investor, author, philanthropist, and humanitarian. He is best known as the principal founder of Microsoft Corporation. And so it shouldn't be a surprise to know that Bill Gates has always loved to code; he was a computer "non-geek" from the get go! In fact, he began writing and developing software while still a teenager! Now look at him today! Because he focused on pursuing what was a truly authentic passion for himself, aligned with his true being, he became the youngest billionaire and the wealthiest person on the planet at the age of 31! And his company's success is largely attributed to his ability to come up with ideas for his team to develop software much like Michael Jackson used to put out songs. If he didn't love what he was doing, this wouldn't be possible!

Now, that's <u>Authentic Power</u> created from a truly **<u>Kicka$$ Happy</u>** Place!

Oprah Winfrey is a talk show host, media executive, actress, billionaire philanthropist, and undoubtedly one of the biggest thought leaders of modern times. She began reading at 3 years old and reciting soon after with an innate love for delivering devotions. In fact, in her early years, she lived on a sprawling farm and spent many an hour preaching to the animals and her corn cob doll. Today, it is her warm-hearted, open personal style that has attracted millions of followers all over the World. She is on the level and real, and people love that. Furthermore, she has refused to compromise her personal integrity for the bottom line. Needless to say, the bottom line has continued to grow exponentially as a natural byproduct of her ability to confidently and courageously, stand up, again and again, for what she believes in. And it is in her desire to serve with a compassionate heart that brings her great fulfillment AND **<u>Kicka$$ Happyness</u>**!

J. Cole is a well-known spiritually conscious rapper, singer, songwriter, and record producer who continues to give people what HE wants, and not what is expected of him. He has won many prestigious Hip Hop awards including "Top Rap Album", and "Most Impact" with his song, "Crooked Smile", about basically loving ourselves as we are. He remains an independent artist with the freedom to speak his truth in a way that has had a powerfully positive impact on the music industry. And I would imagine that passionately sharing what he loves naturally produces within him, an elevated state of **Kicka$$ Happyness!**

What do these famous people have in common? They didn't chase money. They fostered their passion. They developed an innate gift that allowed them to produce with ease with richly abundant financial rewards as a natural outcome. They weren't worried about what others thought. They were willing to be vulnerable, to share their most private beliefs. They were willing to step away from external control and to embrace their own <u>Power</u> by <u>Authentically</u> showing up, again and again! They created from their **<u>"Happy Space"</u>**, aligned with Source/God which is ALWAYS energy-rich in nature!

Now, you may be really good at a lot of things, especially if you've been trained. However, unless you are passionate about what you're doing, you will never be as good as you could be which is way better than good. This would show up more like extraordinarily talented!

For example, I found that I was a great classroom teacher with a solid reputation for helping to make a positive impact in most of the students' lives. However, it got to a point, where I felt restless and unfulfilled. I wanted to make an even greater impact, and to have more freedom to create the programs and curricula that I believed could potentially produce dramatic and long-lasting results for the students. And although I made up a lot of silly and fun poems in my teaching career, it was nowhere at the level of which I was capable. I had to step out of the mundane to step into the insane way that life could truly show up for me.

Today, I am a catalyst for others to develop their own Authentic Power (created in their **"Happy Space"**) through collaborative, creative projects that promote positive self-expression. The operative word here is "collaborative". You see, I have mentored many young emcees who want to be the next big rapper with their name plastered all over billboards, writing number one hits, and owning fancy cars. And to be completely transparent, at one time, that was me, too, dipped just a bit too deep in my own individual, walled up ego "trance dance" with myself! Fortunately, I applied exactly what I'm encouraging you to do in this book. I checked in with my breath a lot more. Basically, I was able to hip check my anxiety against my old bored way of doing things, and it just naturally melted away under the Zamboni of my dreams, streamed in on my breath!

And what are those dreams you might ask? My dreams, my VISION, is to help especially teens and young people to collectively and consciously create on a level not yet seen in the mainstream! I envision the "We are the World" type of songs AND albums, becoming the norm, with a chorus of voices of all ages coming together to create an amplified synergy of unity. I imagine Beyonce's 2018 Coachella performance duplicated a thousand times over across all demographics. I visualize anthologies from a variety of artistic mediums becoming much more commonplace, with individuals contributing to a collective project that reflects a true sense of community in its production. Most importantly, I envision a global community of **Happy, Happy** People empowering others to find their own <u>Authentic **Happy** Place.</u>

And therein lies MY <u>Authentic Power</u>: using my passion for music and creative expression combined with my deep desire to usher in greater harmony in the World to continue to spark the Evolution of mankind.

Now, it's your turn! What truly turns you on? What desire, besides sex (!!!!) lights up passionately inside you? Is it something you would still do whether or not anyone were ever watching? Does it bring you joy? Do you realize how it might be utilized to empower and inspire others without necessarily having to feed your ego? Is it completely aligned with who YOU ARE? To make sure, check yourself, check yourself, check, check, check yourself, always, to ensure that what you are passionately bringing into the World, you are also *compassionately* bringing into the World. In other words, is it for your benefit only or does it provide value to others? You see, I believe, to feed your soul, you must also feed the souls of others!

Major Action Step:

What are you truly passionate about? What is something you'd do all day, every day, if you could?

Once you've identified it, practice it every day for the next 21 days for at least 1 hour/day.

CHAPTER 4

Speak Life into the
Life You Envision for Yourself!
Recreate Empowering Thought Patterns

"As a man thinketh (in his heart), so is he."
-Book of Proverbs, Chapter 23, verse 7

"Our thoughts create our reality."
-Joe Dispenza

"Our most dominant thought patterns determine how the World shows up for us."
-Mama G

By this time, I am sure you have heard the phrase, "You are what you think." There have been countless prophets, a multitude of references in a variety of books dating back decades and centuries, and a mainstream "buzz" in more recent years about the power of our thoughts. In fact, James Allen's book, As a Man Thinketh, first published back in 1903, has continued to be wildly popular. And thanks to emboldened scientists like Albert Einstein, Bruce Lipton, Gregg Braden and Joe Dispenza, to name just a few, there has been a plethora of scientific experiments to add increasing validity to this basic premise. "We are, in fact, what we think!"

And so how does it actually work? How is it possible? Well, first, I'd like you to think about what we have discovered and accomplished in the last 100 years that seemed absolutely impossible to many at one time. To begin, back in 1920, the idea of a World Wide Network that would connect us to information at our fingertips, in an instant, was inconceivable. In fact, the internet as we know it today, was not officially birthed until 1990. That's a mere 30 years ago. Before then, research was done in libraries, by talking to live witnesses, and with the use of books and encyclopedias. It required an exhaustive amount of time and work compared to Today. And virtual assistances such as Siri and Alexa were non-existent!

Here are some other advances we have made in the last 100 years that at one time appeared to be outside the realm of possibility which, by the way, doesn't exist, unless it's a realm within our own mind that believes it does. I, personally, have come to believe that "Anything is Possible."

1.   Developing handheld computers
2.   Traveling at Supersonic Speeds
3.   Traveling to the moon
4.   Cooking a potato in 10 minutes versus 60 minutes
5.   Recharging batteries
6.   Performing laser therapy
7.   Using artificial limbs
8.   Designing electric wheelchairs
9.   Hiring Virtual Assistants

10.   Running a 4 minute mile
11.   Jumping with a vertical leap of 63.5 inches
       (that's well over 5 feet!)
12.   Having over a thousand billionaires in the World
13.   Being able to predict the path of Hurricanes
14.   Swearing into Office a Black president
15.   Holding the breath for 22 minutes and 22 seconds!
16.   Desegregating schools
17.   Abolishing Apartheid in South Africa
18.   Having goods delivered and paid for while never leaving
       the house.
19.   Manufacturing electric cars
20.   Producing jetpack prototypes

Why such an extensive list? Because I want to remind you of all the amazing discoveries, accomplishments, and advances that have taken place in just the last 100 years that, once again, at one time, appeared to seem impossible.

And so, how did these come about? Well, there's actually a scientific formula with a spiritual component that explains how all of the above was made possible! It goes back to our thoughts, what we think, and what we think we believe!

You see, there had to be someone, somewhere, who thought each of the above was possible! This is where "belief" comes in.

When one imagines a new possibility and begins to believe wholeheartedly without any doubt whatsoever in it coming to fruition, then this begins the germination of it coming to life, literally!

It's like planting a seed with our thought, watering it with our elevated emotions, and providing it with warmth through our ongoing, passionate and focused actions.

Hmmm...this sounds awfully familiar. That's because it's been said a thousand times in a thousand ways by thousands and thousands throughout the ages! It's basically the Law of Attraction, the most Senior Scientific Law that exists in our Universe. And it exists with absolute precision, like any other universal law, whether we believe in it or not! It's like the law of gravity. Every object in the Universe, no matter how great or small, has gravitational pull, because absolutely everything in the Universe vibrates. This vibration helps to create an electromagnetic field around each "object" which contributes to the pull and the push of all objects with respect to each other. And this includes our thoughts! Yes, our thoughts! To help you to understand how this could be, I want you to think of your thoughts as energy packets that carry a particular frequency based on what you're thinking AND what you're feeling about what you're thinking! This energy then interacts with what has been identified as a Universal Field of Consciousness (also known as the Divine Matrix, the Source Field, the Quantum Field, or GOD) that then responds to the energy of the thoughts you put out!

It's like a supercomputer that you are programming to get the output that you desire. And so what is it that you want the output to be?

Do you see yourself happier than you could have ever imagined? Do you see yourself standing in your own power? Are you speaking your own truth? Are you speaking with greater ease and more grace in a way that is more readily received by others? Are you able to witness yourself confidently and courageously Being, WHO YOU ARE, AS YOU ARE, without any fear of judgement? Do you show up as loving and kind? Is yours a life of luxury? Do you imagine meaningful relationships in your life with loyal and honest friends? Do you visualize truly not caring about what anyone thinks about how you dress, how you style your hair, how you act, talk, walk and think? Perhaps you believe you are going to become a famous scientist or doctor or entertainer or athlete.

Here's the deal: if you can conceive it, believe it, and are willing to retrieve it as a potential that already exists, then you can achieve it.

Through your clear intentions coupled with your emotions of gratitude, excitement, love, and appreciation, you can attain more and more expansive goals for a life that sees you Transforming to the Greatness that is already inside of you! Unleash this Divine Power through a mind aligned with the Divine, and watch what shows up! You will blow up! (Figuratively, not literally, of course!)

How do I know this works? Because I've applied it time and time again, and I have become increasingly amazed at how my life has changed.

To begin, I used to be extremely negative. The words that came out of my mouth heard me complain about what seemed to be even the most trivial of circumstances. I constantly spoke about how much physical pain I was in, how angry and frustrated I was, how "sick" of things I was, and guess what? I was confronted with more and more situations for me to choose to be angry and in pain or not. I became sick quite often, and I was a generally miserable person who distracted myself in many ways, putting on a great act with what I thought was a genuine smile, until I crashed and burned under the weight of my own illusion. Basically, I was a Mama with trauma, feeding off the drama of depressed thoughts and suppressed pain that saw, as I mentioned, more and more of the "against the grain" type of experiences show up in my life. Fortunately for me, I finally ended up in the break down lane and was at last willing to accept some roadside assistance.

It led me to the AAA of *Accountability, Awareness, and Authenticity*. First, I had to take responsibility for my life AND the future I desired to create. Second, I had to bravely delve deeper within myself to develop the awareness of how I was actually perpetuating a life of constant struggle and heartache. Finally, I had to choose to grow and expand by persevering through what seemed at times, insurmountable obstacles, in order to reach a level of **personal transformation** that would permit me to unleash my Greatness to the World, and to be **HAPPY** doing it!

In a few words, I had to change my THOUGHTS! You see, our thoughts become words, which then become actions. And my thoughts were producing words and actions... AND reactions that were simply not favorable to my overall well-being and to the well-being of those around me.

I literally had to learn to think and to speak differently if I wanted to be **HAPPY!**

For example,

1. ~~I am in pain~~.
   Instead, I am developing more ease and comfort in my body.

2. ~~I am so unfocused~~.
   Instead, I am mastering the art of laser sharp, task-oriented focus.

3. ~~Everybody seems to fall out of love with me~~.
   Instead, I am learning to fall deeply in love with myself.

Now, why does it matter how we phrase our statements?

It matters, because, first of all, there is a negative perspective and a more positive perspective. Secondly, they each carry a different energy frequency. One carries a lower vibration (negative perspective) while the other carries a higher vibration (positive perspective). One feels heavy and more dense while the higher vibration feels lighter and more free. In fact, Dr. Masaru Emoto, a Japanese scientist and healer, authored various books on water, demonstrating how our thoughts and our vibes can affect crystal formation in water.

Basically, he filled up 100 petri dishes with water. He spoke hateful, harmful words and phrases to 50% of these dishes for a period of 3 days. At the same time, he spoke words of love and praise to the other 50%. At the end of the 3 days, the water in the petri dishes to which Dr. Emoto spoke lovingly displayed, beautiful, intricate, coherent water crystals. The "hated on" water, however, formed misshaped crystals that appeared muddled and dark in appearance.

Now, I'd like to remind you that we are made up of about 60% water. So you could imagine how Emoto's experiments might have practical application for the words that we choose to use and to listen to!

To relate this to the Quantum Field, our words transmit the signal (much like a radio frequency to a tower) that shares our request (whether we're aware of it or not) with the Quantum Field. And then it is the quality of our emotions which determine how weak or strong the signal becomes. For example, an angry person who shouts very strongly, "People are such a fu***** pain in the a**!" will surely receive precisely just that, more evidence to confirm his or her perception of "his or her" World. On the other hand, "someone who speaks in a way that is less than self-assured, saying, "I think I can be an amazing singer," sends out a confusing, weak signal. For although the statement is positive, it is stated with little confidence and little belief. It is missing the fuel (the power) to get that transmission to where it needs to go! It's like a Ferrari with a dead battery, a beautiful intention with no force behind it to put it into motion.

https://thewellnessenterprise.com/emoto/

What is also important to note, is that the subconscious mind which seems to have a direct line to the Quantum Field, does not seem to understand "negatives". So when we say something like, "I don't want anything to do with cancer," it's not the "don't" that's understood, but the "cancer". It's like hosting a cancer walk where all the focus is on cancer. Ever hear, "where the focus goes is where the energy flows?" Well, that's a real thing, scientifically and unequivocally proven, time and time again!

Instead of Cancer Walks, perhaps it would benefit us to begin "Peak Health Walks". In that same vein, it might be quite advantageous to rename quite a few walks and events:

Perhaps, "Suicide Prevention" events can be replaced with "In the Name of Self-love" events; "A March for Hunger" replaced with "A March for Well-nourished and Satiated"; a "Walk for Autism" replaced with "A Celebration for Neurodiversity".

Do you see what I'm getting at? We could either dwell on our pain and our struggle and what we don't want, and it will continue to persist, or we could empower ourselves by focusing on what it is we DO want.

To practice putting yourself in the habit of this, I would invite you to consider listening to Abraham Hicks as channeled by Esther Hicks. All you have to do is Google Abraham and Esther Hicks, and a multitude of helpful videos will pop up!

Major Action Step:

Every time you catch yourself making a negative statement or comment, stop and take the time to rephrase it to focus on a favorable outcome.

Ex. ~~I'm so tired all the time. I have no energy.~~
I am working on increasing my vitality.

See Appendix C for a list of valuable resources on the Power of Our Thoughts.

CHAPTER 5

Allow Nature to Be Your Teacher
Unsubscribe From the Grind Mentality

"Look at a tree, a flower, a plant. Let your awareness rest upon it. How still they are, how deeply rooted in Being."
-Eckhart Tolle

"Patience is the sleepy, star-filled night which blankets itself in reassurance as it waits for the first glimpses of dawn to creep in."
– Mama G

"It is the daily rhythm of the sea's surf, of our beating heart, and our inbreaths and outbreaths that remind us to maintain a balance of productivity and receptivity."
-Mama G

How often have you heard, "You must hustle and work hard, and basically grind, grind, grind, if you want to be successful"? I'm sure many, many times. I know I have. And you know what? I believed it at one time, even though it didn't make sense. For example, I allowed myself the liberty of 3 months to do absolutely nothing after the death of my partner. During that time period, I would heavily meditate on plants and trees and flowers. I participated in much deep self-reflection, like that mentioned in chapter 2, and because of my receptive, deeply relaxed state, I witnessed the most amazing events. I once saw a bud spontaneously blossom right in front of my eyes! I also regularly interacted with plants and watched as the leaves quivered. I even saw what I understood to be "angelic sparks" above my then 6 year old daughter's head when she sought my comfort at night (*Remember, she had just lost a parent to cancer.) This receptive phase helped me to find the magic in life once again and to renew my faith in a Benevolent Divine Being.

However, after that 3 month period, when my "family leave act" was up, I felt the NEED to figure out my life, and to begin to take action! I didn't want to be perceived as lazy! Imagine that! I had just spent 3 ½ years as a caretaker while working full-time and raising 2 young children, had averaged less than 5 hours a night's sleep during that time period, was under extreme stress, losing 10 pounds on an already light frame, and had even experienced 2 panic attacks. On top of that, just one week after my partner's funeral where I watched my then 9 year old son help to carry the casket, I found evidence that my partner had had a 20 year affair that produced a child. Bring on Jerry Springer! Now, in hindsight, I understand how I helped to contribute to this circumstance. I truly believe it was a co-created reality and one of the many gifts that have been bestowed upon me in this life, so that I could fuel my future with sky-rocketing desires!

 However, as a human living a human experience, let's just say, if I had not succumbed to the mainstream, "work, work, work, push through" mentality, that I probably would have felt more relaxed in taking the time to heal without putting pressure on myself to be more productive and to aggressively earn the money to take care of my family. I have only sporadically worked full-time since the death of my partner 10 years ago, yet it wasn't until just recently that I felt free to fully rest when I was not in a place to effectively execute my dreams.

In fact, it was this "grind mentality" that led me to a few "shake ups" or what many refer to as a "wake up call". The "highly active, on the go, hyper mode, and needing to slow... down, quite a bit" me, was literally taken out by the Universe. The Universe spoke very loudly and clearly around the time I was driving for Uber as a way to fund my dreams while working around my children's schedules. It happened while playing basketball with my teen son in the backyard. After he sealed a win with a formidable dunk, the once overly competitive me that should have called it quits after 2 games, fell hard. In fact, my injury was so bad, I was unable to even sit up. I was in excruciating pain as my left foot hung by what seemed like the tiniest of tethers. This was serious. My children brought me a blanket to lie on, water to hydrate myself, lots of ice, and even an umbrella to shade me from the noon day, summer sun. It would be hours before I felt confident enough to crawl back into the house without fear of completely snapping off my foot!

Now, at this time, I had no health insurance, so I resorted to the multitude of natural healing modalities I had learned after I left my teaching job years earlier. I performed energy work on myself, and had no choice, but to completely and fully rest. It was time for a "forced" receptive mode after overly aggressive, non-productivity.

The blessing from this Divinely imposed respite saw **2 books of poetry** spontaneously blossom from my now fully present creative space.

Interestingly enough, these poems were about nature. One entitled: Nature's Lessons: *What the World is Trying to Teach Us*, the second, Nature's Essence: *How the Divine Expresses Itself*. These books were written in a mere 2 days as I lay prone in my backyard, with what would be the beginning of a 4 year recovery.

Since then, the teacher who used to show up with serious bronchial coughs, weeks of laryngitis, and sometimes, low grade fevers, realized the importance of taking the time to rest. For there is no such thing as a productive grind, in my opinion, or at least an efficient one. For example, what would happen to our tide pools that teem with wildlife as an integral part of an oceanside ecosystem if an area were to experience only high tide? What would happen if night followed night, day followed day, if an inbreath never saw an outbreath? What would happen if we produced, produced, yet didn't take the time to prepare and to plan? What would happen if we talked and never listened, listened and never talked? I believe you get the point I'm making here. Nature quite wondrously demonstrates in so many ways, I believe, just how important it is to have balance in our lives.

And so let us do just that! Let us follow the lead of our greatest teacher, and learn to create, to produce, to execute, and to flourish with the greatest of ease and with the greatest of grace. Let us be both passionate and supportive, both content-focused and execution-driven,
both imaginative and functional, both determined and
gentle, both confident and humble, both active and still.

Let us BE. Let us DO. Let us BE. Let us DO. Let us BE.

Major Action Step:

What is one way you can bring more balance into your life, so that you always show up at your best and fully present?

CHAPTER 6

Take Time to Purge!
Design Space for a new wardrobe, a new home, new friendships, a new outlook...

"A man is rich in proportion to the number of things he can afford to let alone."- **Henry David Thoreau**

"As you let go of the complications, emotional toxins, and everything else that isn't serving you, you will be free to experience the happiness that exists in simplicity."
– Deepak Chopra

"Simplify your life, and watch the true beauty of life present itself in its ever present glory."
-Mama G

Purge!!!! Blaaaah! Let it all go, like you just had a drunken-filled, deeply regrettable, inebriated evening, and you want it to be a very distant memory! Yes, let it ALL go! If you truly want to start anew and to claim the type of intensely <u>transformative power</u> that exists within your very Being, then let it all go. And do it NOW! Not tomorrow, not next week, TODAY. Begin TODAY, and continue, until you begin to feel lighter and freer than you have ever felt in your entire life.

"Well, sounds great," you might say to yourself, "but what are we letting go of? The chewed up sock my dog has been carrying around for the last 8 months, the jeans I wore 20 years ago during my clubbing days, my high school yearbook, my last dye job, my duct-taped sneakers?"

Yes, yes, and YEEES, all of it! And trust that you will be way better than okay and on your way to better days with better ways! BETTER, BETTER, BETTER, than EVAH! "How so," you shoot back, "when it seems like I'm giving up so much?" Okay, I get it. I've been there, too. It's difficult to donate those jeans to someone who could really, really use them when you hold on to the false hope that you just might fit into those jeans again someday. Honestly though, would you wear those jeans anyway if they fit you, 20 years and multiple trends later? You see, simply holding onto those jeans is evidence of just how outdated your beliefs may have become. Could you imagine a 20 year old with a onesie tucked into the recesses of his/her closet with the hope of one day fitting into it again? Seriously, it's basically coming from the same fear-based mindset that desperately seeks approval from the External World. Like, look at me! I must be amazing and special, because I've had the willpower and the control to keep the weight off. What it's really saying is, "I'm afraid to change. I'm afraid of the unknown. I'm afraid of losing control of a future that is uncertain. I need others to love me, to tell me how special I am. It is frightening to let go of an Identity that's become familiar and comfortable for me."

The jeans become a fallback, a safety net, a symbol of what it means to truly change. Change might mean the jeans become ripped, stained, even shredded to pieces as you struggle to overcome the challenges that await your journey of deep

<u>transformation.</u> No one ever said it would be easy. However, it can be very much simplified!

Start by reducing the clutter in your physical environment. Donate the canned food you haven't touched in months, along with the 10 extra plate settings you've never used, the variety of mismatched coffee mugs collecting dust in the cabinet above your refrigerator, and the sleeping bags you're saving for the "someday" camping trip. Then sift through your closet (or closets!) and donate as many articles of clothing you own, to the point where it feels uncomfortable, including the shoes! The shoes, too. You're not the Queen of Sheba, unless you are.

Then walk away from toxic relationships, try a new hairstyle, a new hair color, reassess your living situation, your job, your attitude, your routines, everything!!!

Make it a daily practice, and it will surely become less painful and actually rather fun! I mean that! When we let go of anything, we create space for something new and exciting. It makes life an adventure, and that can be quite fun, if we just allow ourselves to accept a level of uncertainty in our lives.

To begin, doesn't it feel great to wear new clothes? It's like a new personality is showing up. You look different. You feel different. And it often feels fresh and rewarding. You can choose new styles and new colors, and finally stop trying to fit into those 20 year old jeans, for goodness sake!

You might also paint your room...a different color, of course. My parents have painted their house many, many times in the 40 plus years they have lived in their house.

Guess what color it was when they bought it? Guess what color they repainted it, every single time? You guessed it, the same color. I suggest you choose a new color that matches the new YOU that you are becoming!

Keep going! Don't stop! How about redecorating the house, rearranging the furniture, replacing your bedspread? Redesign your life in any way you can, and feel exhilarated by the newness which is your new personal reality showing up just as you have desired! You are the creator, if you choose!

Now, I wouldn't ask you to go full throttle if I wasn't willing to do the same, especially since I KNOW that if you picked up this book, you aren't looking for cookie crumbs. You want the super-sized, just out of the oven, mouth-watering chocolate chip cookie of transformations. So take a big bite, and be excited about it! After all, you're letting go of the musty, dusty you and cleaning out the cobwebs of your mind that is now ready to shine with a new glory. You are no longer traumatized, feeling victimized and stuck in old neural patterns. You will not sit on a couch, complacent and achingly adjacent to another gallon of ice cream you just devoured to fill the void that all the clutter in the World could never fill.

You no longer have to wistfully watch your children spend more and more time away from home, creating and living their own life. It's actually a gift, because that empty nest now opens you up to the whole limitless sky of possibilities! And what's a life without possibilities?

It's like cleaning out that refrigerator at the end of the week, with a fresh, sparkly look, so that you can refill it with new surprises for the upcoming week. Maybe it's salmon with a honey glaze and a side of fresh spinach versus the frozen nuggets you ate last week. Perhaps a decadent dessert to salaciously savor versus just another sleeve of crème-filled cookies. Or how about freshly squeezed orange juice versus the heavily concentrated clutter in your home and in your mind?

Guess what?! I've tasted the salmon! I've indulged in the decadent dessert! And I've thoroughly enjoyed the freshly squeezed orange juice. Beyond that, I've been able to check off multiple items on my bucket list in a very short period of time, simply by "cleaning house"! Now, I want you to understand that "cleaning house" is an ongoing process just like cleaning out your refrigerator. Imagine if you only cleaned out your refrigerator once in a lifetime?? Oh, my, I don't think there'd be enough baking soda to manage that one! Furthermore, it would severely limit your options.

For me personally, I'm all about exponentially expanding my options! At one time, I owned 2 outfits and slept on a mattress in a corner in my living room. Why? So I could rent out my room and have the time I desired to work on my dream life. I also wanted to be able to continue to support my family as a single mom, both financially and in the added time I'd be able to invest in them, however that might have looked.

My most recent "cleaning house" was a MAJOR space creator, in every way! After moving to Tampa from the Boston area in 2017, I spent 2 years confronting more challenges than some confront in a lifetime. In fact, arriving in our new home just days before the arrival of Hurricane Irma seemed to have been a very clear warning of what lay ahead! And so 2 years later, after intense personal and financial struggle, I decided it was time for another fresh start!

And so I began by selling a few select items and donating the rest. The plan was to move into a luxury apartment near the beach in Miami. However, I was not yet sure whether or not we'd be fortunate enough to find one that was furnished. TRUST. There was no way I was taking anything with me, except perhaps the clothes on my back. And I essentially did just that. I unloaded all my clothes and shoes and literally packed a carry on with what I had left. Following my lead, my teenage daughter filled bags and bags to bring over to the Salvation Army. My son was away at college, so we opted to put his items into storage.

Then came the car, a 2011 Honda Civic Hybrid that had about 120,000 miles and was in need of more work. Easy. I attempted to sell it to a dealer, yet the sales team appeared greedy. So I donated that, too, and helped a struggling family with a car they desperately wanted and which they graciously received! Next, I rented a U-Haul, and just weeks after our decision to move, we arrived in South Beach to begin our new life in a completely furnished, spacious, 2-bedroom luxury condominium.

We began enjoying all the amazing amenities right away! This included an infinity pool, a fitness studio, a sauna, and a hot tub. We also began to frequent the beach, located just 2 blocks from our complex, as well as the Bay, with casual walks from time to time. To continue, we were assigned 2 parking spots in a secure garage and our surroundings were lavish. However, we knew we hit the bulls-eye, when we started to encounter **happy**, heart-centered people every day.

Now, please understand that it was my willingness to change, to let go, to trust, that opened up even more incredible opportunities for my family and me! I paid off all my debt with the sale of the house in Tampa, hired a second business coach, infused more money into my business, provided us with financial security, paid my son's college tuition, bought my daughter and I all new clothes, planned a wonderful family vacation right here on the Beach, and began to write my second book. Most importantly, I just felt **happier** and **happier** at the life I had created!

Now, I am not bragging. I simply want you to understand what is possible for us when we decide to change and to let go, and to move on. And when we make a practice out of it, we become better and better at it. We trust more, and we make our moves more decisively, and life shows up more enticingly!

Still feeling reluctant, perhaps still slightly questioning the validity of what I'm sharing? Well, then let's shift away from my own powerfully personal experience for a few moments and look to our masterful teacher, Mother Nature. Would you doubt her? Would you doubt Father Sky? Would you doubt the absolute grandeur on display, put into place by a most Benevolent Creator? You might, depending on what space you're in right now. I know I did, but evidence has become the loudest voice for me! I believe it can do the same for you!

With that being said, let's begin with the butterfly. It takes flight in all its gloriously majestic grace and never looks back at the shredded chrysalis it just left behind. More specifically, how do you think a Monarch is able to travel thousands of miles from the U.S. to hit up its sweet spot in Southwestern México (to survive the cold North American winter and ensure a food source for survival)? You guessed it. It leaves absolutely all of its baggage behind and freely says hello to FREEDOM!

Yet there's more to the story! It appears that not all Monarch butterflies migrate! I've read that a Monarch born in the beginning of the summer months sticks around and lives an average of only 2-6 weeks. On the other hand, the Monarchs born in late summer, just as Autumn is looming around the corner, automatically head for the border. They hang out for the winter and head back north in the Spring.

It is incredible to think about the vast differences in both the lifespan and the life experience of these groups of Monarchs born just weeks apart! Upon deeper reflection, I would surmise that perhaps those Monarchs born in the beginning of the summer months might become somewhat complacent, having grown accustomed to the ease with how life is showing up for them... La, la, la, la...summer breeze, flit about, breathe and Be, in my simplicity. Hmmmm....beautiful existence, I might add.

Yet, *what if, what if*....there could be more that they could extract from life...more time, more nectar, more freedom? What if they were willing to stick around to brave the increasingly cooler nights, with a new season on the horizon, to which they were willing to adapt? Would they be willing to let go of the life they'd known and even enjoyed? Would they be willing to travel thousands of miles as one of the most fragile creatures created on this planet, to perhaps confront unexpected predators and maybe even some wild weather for the possibility for more? *What if, what if...*

Still want more evidence? Well, there's plenty of it! Mother Nature doesn't mess around. She has shown up well-prepared for our benefit. So leave Google alone right now, and let's step outside to check out more of what she has to offer. Well, well, well, insects abound! These seemingly pesky little nature beings can teach us quite a bit. Like they molt and bolt! They don't stick around wondering if they should hang onto their "armor". They instinctively grow and expand into the next version of themselves. And you don't see them grabbing anyone else's "armor" either. That's a form of perversion that we humans are still figuring out, because somehow we've been given the ability to think. The challenge is we often overthink and forget to check in with our instinct.

In fact, it's the overthinking that creates self-doubt and indecisiveness, allowing just enough time for fear to build an energetic wall around our heart, a low frequency dense armor that can become rather heavy to carry around. In fact, if we allow it to go on for too long, constantly suppressing our desires and our dreams for the most exhilarating life, then we can become chronically depressed, feeling suppressed and oppressed by our own doing!

Now, it is a little known fact that insects are not able to breathe while they molt. Interestingly enough, we often do the same when confronted with the uncertainty of our future. This can and often does translate into anxiety, and for some, even panic attacks. I know. I've been there! And so I highly recommend that you do in fact BREATHE through it all, through all of it!! For breathing is what fuels us; it's what provides us with the Life Force to move forward through all the trepidation and stress-induced excitation. Furthermore, breathing deeply, fully, and completely calms and soothes us. It also precipitates the body's ability to release pain we have most likely subconsciously held onto, almost as if we built a dam within ourselves to avoid a mess!

And what would that mess look like? Well, that beautiful distressed mess could look like you sobbing and slobbering, nose dripping with you belly gripping, next to a box of tissues, blowing and honking! And if that mess becomes you, then I believe you are truly blessed, and it becomes you to be that blessed! It means you pass the test! You exit the grief, and you cannot tell me that doesn't bring relief!

Whew! This is a reminder to revisit what I've shared in chapter 1 many times over, to make it a way of life. I mean that! Why? Because, I believe life is about creating anew in every moment, and in order to do that, we must make letting go and release a part of the process. I absolutely do! Just like the skies cry from time to time to keep the sun shining bright, so must we.

Personally, I trust that I have already experienced my darkest days and my deepest pain. However, I still have a good cry once in a while, sometimes without even knowing why, just because I can feel the heaviness start to build, and it just feels great! To be honest, I had a solid cry just before I wrote this. And the space that I created brought an influx of truly amazing inspiration. I hope you are feeling that right now, for it is Divinely delivered through me to you! So purge, purge, purge, fa, la, la, la...I'm the butterfly....

Wait, what? Still not enough proof? You want more?

Okay, okay, I got you. No worries. Nature has a lot to say, so let's give her a little more of a listen!

"Shhhh....shhhh"....she's asking us to be real quiet for her next guest. Sssssss.......sssssssss......oh my, well, look at what we have here! Satya the snake, already on her 4th take, coming off a very recent "shake and bake", "peel and feel"....the growth!

Woooweee! Hmmm....it appears that Satya is now fit to be a sage. She wishes to do the talking here.

"Thank you for your kind words. Again, I am Satya, and I have experienced many moons in a variety of locales. I am quite unique as you might imagine. Today, I'm feeling quite relaxed, refreshed and rejuvenated after a recent molt. You see, my skin had begun to feel a bit too thick, quite tight, and truthfully, rather restrictive and laboriously limiting. I soon realized that it was time for the next level of transformation in my life that would allow me to grow and to expand. I have always welcomed this expansion and the opportunity for my ever increasing awareness about myself and the World around me to unfold!

And so I wonder, how do you respond when you start to feel closed in, feeling like your choices are limited, feeling like you want more?

Well, if I could be bold enough to share my experience, I would highly recommend letting go of whatever is holding you back. I know you know. The choice to change can be a scary one, to say the least, yet change you must! Think of change as your friend. Much like the change in your pocket, it can add up to an incredibly large amount that you'll be able to cash in one day."

So whaddya say? Time to purge, and then splurge, perhaps?

Yes, indeed, kick it to the curb, so to speak, and let me witness you begin to more courageously step into your <u>Authentic Power</u> as the **<u>Happiest Person</u>** you could have ever imagined!

Major Action Step: Decide what it is you believe you must purge right now to help create the space for something new and exciting! Is it a bag of clothes, saying goodbye to a relationship, replacing a bad habit with a new, empowering one?

CHAPTER 7

Mindfully Switch Up Your Routine
Build Your Mind Power By Firing Up
New Neural Networks

"As your body moves, your brain grooves."
-Jim Kwik

"But you can't change the fruit without changing the root." - Stephen R. Covey

"A 6-pack in mind fitness is going to involve some Intentional practices."
-Mama G

Wow! Congratulations! You're are a Rockin' Superstar, a Super Rock Star, purging left and right, breathing in and out, and doing what you love!

To rocket even higher, like you fired up in a new age socket with the fire in your pockets, you've got to STOP IT! "STOP IT?! Why would I stop now, Mama G? I'm on a finger-lickin', heart-tickin', mind-trippin' roll. Why, after 7 chapters of industriously induced, reproduced co-creativity, would you want me to STOP IT???"

Okay, I get it. Let me clear up the confusion. When I say "STOP IT", I'm referring to the triggers in your life that will undoubtedly keep showing up until you stop working off the old neural networks that cause you to react from outdated circuitry. Basically, I'm talking about the "loopty-doops" that get you loopy and back on the stoop with your shoulders in a droop, because something happens that appears all too reminiscent of a really bad experience you've once had. You see, choosing to remain in these thought patterns that can sadden you is like playing a never-ending game of Russian Roulette. It never really allows the stress to leave the house until you kick out the DJ that keeps playing the same track! And that DJ is you!

Now I say, let's keep the music playing, but switch it up! Let's disengage from the tired, old sh** and make a new playlist. I mean, a completely new playlist. Don't even attempt to mix in those old songs, overplayed where you felt betrayed! Slay those demons right now, and get off that emotional roller coaster. Because it is time to MOVE ON!!

So how do we build the mind power that helps to balance our mood and keeps us in the present moment, enjoying the present moment? How do we extract the wisdom from our past, empower our present, and fuel our future?

Well, let's gravitate back to the mind, body, spirit connection. I call it the Holy Trinity, and just like the sides of an equilateral triangle, they are all equally important. However, lately, it seems like mindset is getting all the glory, all the attention. At one time it was the spirit, and another time, it was the body, so I guess it's only fair that the mindset gets to step up.

But what about the part where some say, "Just be positive. Choose joy. Make your gratitude list. Change your attitude. You can change your mind, right now!"

To me, it was like telling the addictive eater who has become morosely overweight to just drop 30 pounds on the spot or the lifelong atheist to just accept that there is a Supreme Being on which we can lean.

"Arrrgggggh!" I used to often exclaim to myself! Honestly, what I used to say was much worse than that; however, this is a PG book. ☺

Guess what?? As someone who once experienced very intense, ongoing trauma, as someone who was literally in the grip of death hundreds of times over, it wasn't that easy to just be positive!!!! In fact, it was painfully humiliating and infuriating to me that I was not yet able to just be positive. Heck, I had spent a lifetime being negative, had developed deeply rooted Oak Tree type thinking, behaving, and acting. How could I just be positive? Have you ever tried to dig up a full-grown tree by its roots?

It's close to impossible, and definitely not something I believe we could ever do on our own. I needed help, a lot of help! I needed a bulldozer to move the crap, a front loader to scoop it up, and a dump truck to haul it away! Now, I could have just popped a few pills on a daily and slept walked through the rest of my life. I suppose I could have also opted for a lobotomy. Yet, as negative as I once thought, even that seemed a bit extreme, like another bad dream that I didn't want to be a part of.

And so I switched up the routine of going to doctors who only seemed to be concerned about the symptoms of both my physical and emotional pain without addressing the root cause. I walked away from the medical establishment with chronic UTIs, painful and uncomfortable arthritis, recurring migraine headaches, digestive issues, tenderness in my breasts, and a generally depressed state of mind. I then honored myself by working with powerful healers who were able to access the Cosmos in a way that promoted the integration of every angle of that equilateral triangle. It was as if the greatest scientist, the greatest spiritual leader and the greatest doctor all showed up to collaborate and to infuse their individual strengths for a ramped up, synergistic profound healing that each would never have been able to do on their own.

Even navigation requires at the very least, a longitude and a latitude working in tandem to target a location.

Anyway, as a result, 10 years later, I no longer experience any of those symptoms. Not one pill, not one surgery, not one protocol. I did it all naturally.

Now, clearly, there were other changes that had to be made to begin to align my mind and my way of thinking along a more positive frame of reference.

I began to change more habits. For example, I no longer drank even socially as wine, which I absolutely loved with Italian food, was too acidic for my already acidic, sometimes sadistic, mind. Of course, I also cut out most Italian food. I opted not to eat bread or pasta, and to consciously eat more fresh fruits and vegetables, less meat. The real "kicker" in the pants, however, was sugar.

Refined, processed, completely void of nutrients, sugar! I had been an addict for YEARS, and it took me that long to realize just how damaging sugar can be to the body!

Sugar offers absolutely no nutritive value to the body. Even worse, it BLOCKS the nutrients from healthy foods from being absorbed! It acts like a bully standing between you and the gate to the carnival. You're looking for a great time, but instead you walk away disappointed and fatigued from your multiple efforts at creating the energy required to feel excited about life! In a sense, sugar, especially in large amounts, can be a literal mood killer...a buzz kill!

Because I'm not into "Buzz Kills", I essentially had to learn how to become "high" on life. I changed more habits. I began practicing yoga regularly, and soon after, added daily meditation to my pre-breakfast menu. I spent even more time in nature and absorbed the healthy ions found outside. I literally began to hug trees and caress leaves, I kid you not! It began to bring me greater and greater joy, much more than another night sitting on the couch watching movies. I began to walk before the sun rose. I basked in the pre-dawn energy and marveled at the wildlife that came alive at this time, the wildlife that had been mysteriously non-existent on my previous walks. Fawns stood sweetly on the side of the road, foxes skittered across the street, raccoons sauntered around roadside trees, bunny rabbits perched themselves on lawns, skunks stealthily slunk by me, possum scurried along, and the birds began their gentle chorus of chirps. And I, I began to learn to breathe in the essence of life.

And the more I tapped into what I believe to be the true nature of our existence, the easier it became for me to change more habits and to expedite my healing. I grew and expanded in ways I never thought possible!

Once I saw the positive effects of my transformation, it encouraged me to want more! It was like I found the initial spark that flamed my renewed passion for life, and I wanted to continue to fuel that fire! Each new, more healthy habit was like a fat log added to an already roaring campfire.

And to keep that rip roaring fire with desire, efficiently wired in my brain, I made even small, seemingly trivial changes to my daily non-routine. As a "righty", I began brushing my teeth with my left hand. In fact, I began to use my left hand for many tasks. I consciously paid attention to how I dressed and switched it up. For example, if I appeared to be in the habit of putting on both my socks before my sneakers, I would put one sock and one sneaker on before moving to the other foot and doing the same. I would move through my home, taking a different route as often as I could. This helped to increase my brain power. I was no longer on automatic. In fact, I was taking hold of the wheel, and I was NOW in charge!

I would decide where to go, what to do and how to get there. I was quite literally, in a new groove with nothing to prove! At the risk of sounding new age cliché, I was creating my new reality! Interestingly enough, it was a skill I could work at and improve, like going from a Pee Wee Baller to a Dunk Master!

And so I did just that! I discovered Jim Kwik, CEO of Kwik Learning, and a Master at hacking into our Super brain! He suffered a brain injury as a child, and instead of succumbing to possible limitations with regard to his overall brain functioning, he developed powerful techniques to become an expert in speed-reading, memory improvement, accelerated learning and overall brain performance. By watching his YouTube videos, I became much less reliant on my phone. I began to memorize shopping lists, lock down bullet points for my speeches that I remembered with greater ease, and began to navigate without my cell phone!

In fact, much to the disgust of my teen children, I prefer to ask a live person for directions when I believe I can make the time to do so. This not only helps to produce more brain cells; it allows me to connect with more people! And in turn, it helps to elevate my mood. And I believe it could do the same for you!

Remember the equilateral triangle? Mind, Body, Spirit? The simple task of switching up basic routines addresses the physiology, as new habits perpetuate the production of new, neural networks. These, in turn, help to maximize our mental power with the ability to identify more possibilities from a greater perspective, which in turn, empowers us and uplifts our spirit. We begin to believe in the process, the connection, the outcome; and we naturally want more!

Major Action Step: What is one simple task that you can do differently and consistently, every day, that will help to create a new neural network in your brain and thus strengthen your mind power?!

CHAPTER 8

Learn to Value Yourself
Invest in Yourself and Stand in Your Power

"To double your net worth, double your self-worth. Because you will never exceed the height of your self-image." -Robin Sharma

"Your most important sale is to sell yourself to yourself." - Maxwell Maltz

"Taking complete ownership of your own unique gifts that have the potential to bring tremendous value to others is like a powerful SEO that allows you to stand out, like a burst of sunshine on an otherwise gloomy day." -Mama G

Dang, after the bang, bang, bang of frustrated fists on many a wall, door, table, or any other hard surface, we can only begin to turn the tide of tyranny on our own self-worth by beginning to first, recognize our own beauty. Trust me, this one is a doozy, I truly believe! This is especially true if we've ever experienced any type of trauma that has us doubting the love that forever courses through our very being from what I know to be an incredibly compassionate, loving Source. To be honest, it is sometimes not enough to have two loving supportive parents and a more or less happy home when tragedy strikes from somewhere else. Sometimes it's a dangerously dictated disability that impedes our capacity to perceive the beauty in the atypical way we've shown up. Sometimes it's ongoing abuse where we unfortunately get used to being the short end of somebody else's fuse. Sometimes it's the sudden and tragic death of a family member, friend, or colleague. Sometimes it's the hope for a seemingly positive outcome when our expectations have been catastrophically crushed.

Whatever the reason, trauma can stifle us in moving beyond even the most trifle events in our life. It often becomes a tortuous, twisted journey, riddled with fears, doubts, and insecurities, much like the way potholes show up after an intense winter storm. Unbeknownst to us, we almost immediately begin to question the meaning of life, its purpose, and whether or not we have any real significance. We become worrisome, walled up overthinkers who contemplate the vastness of the Universe as a backdrop of demonic darkness that could care less about the "tiny worthless speck of an existence" we seem to be.

We begin with outraged outbursts, demanding answers. WHY? WHY ME? WHY IS THIS HAPPENING? WHAT DID I DO TO DESERVE THIS? WHAT KIND OF GOD WOULD ALLOW THIS?! I HATE MY LIFE! GOD IS A JOKE!

Wow...that's some spewing what's been brewing for much too long. And it's not usually our cup of tea!

Even worse, however, once we move past the initial shock, we maintain a careless whisper that can last for months and even years. We ever so quietly and maybe not so quietly, at times, tell ourselves that we're not enough. We're not worth anyone sticking around, not even God (or any Supreme Being that has our back). We compare ourselves to others, we judge others, we point out our imperfections, we worry about what others think, we believe we must overdo, overproduce, we attach ourselves to multiple social media platforms with a focus on vanity metrics, and we complain about the way life keeps showing up for us...exactly the way we think it will!

You see, after the trauma, we often bring in the Drama through the Denial of and the Distraction from Deep pain and struggle. I call that a "D" in life, because it usually leads us to another "D", absolute, aching Despair, with our Soul in need of some respite and repair.

And so to begin to reunite the fragmented pieces of our spirit, we must continue to practice and remember everything I've mentioned in this book, thus far. We must take the time to heal. We must take the time to reflect and to connect. We must focus on that which we do well. We must become more mindful about the thoughts we entertain and the words we speak. We must allow nature to become one of our greatest teachers. We must be willing to purge, to let go, of physical clutter, mental chatter, and embrace spiritual matters. We must be willing to change our habits, in all forms, bit by bit. And we must do this, step by step, with a forward progression, sometimes backward regression, yet with the intention of always moving forward.

The great news is there's always more we can do, more we can put into place and more we can practice, as a way to confidently and courageously extend our amazingness to the World!

I call it the "two-fold, bring me the gold, that's what's happening" path back to worthiness. I liken it to a wonderful walk along Dorothy's Yellow Brick Road (from the Wizard of Oz) that culminates in the self-realization of the Divine Power within ourselves to create whatever it is we want to BE in our life.

Number One: INVEST IN YOURSELF.

In fact, invest in yourself FIRST, ALWAYS... physically, financially, mentally, emotionally, and spiritually. Recognize that you, you, and YOU deserve the best of the best of the best at ALL times.

The "FIRST" part is a critical component in learning to feel captivated by yourself☺ Think about it. Self-love and self-care show up as really sexy. Why? Because it's the attractive person who is dressed neatly, cleaned up, well-groomed and manicured, light on their feet and looking well-rested that values him or herself enough to do and be all that.

On the other hand, it seems fairly easy to identify that person who does not necessarily hold him or herself in high regard. This is often evidenced by wrinkly, worn, sometimes slightly stained clothing, perhaps unkempt hair or hair hastily tucked in a ponytail (for men, an unintended 3 day stubble), a tight-lipped neutral expression, all with often a shuffle in the step. In fact, it's as if dragging one's feet is the heavy load of emotional baggage that has no room for what could be a sack full of gold coins.

For further emphasis, let me ask you this: If we were to compare self-worth to money, which would you prefer, a crisp, brand new $100 bill, hot off the treasury printing press, or a crumpled and dirty old dollar bill thrust into the corner of an abandoned warehouse?

Let's face it. Nobody wants the "I'll settle for seconds, too busy on the grind to take the time to realign" person who devalues herself.

I know, because, once again, that was me. I felt I had to work hard to prove myself, to show that I was a hard worker. I wasn't lazy. I wasn't a freeloader. I could stand on my own feet. Except I couldn't. I was too worn out. I kept myself busy for the sake of others' seemingly watchful eye (which was really in my own mind) that feared their judgement. I was busy, busy, busy, yet not necessarily productive. I didn't take the time to plan my week, nor to organize my day. My focus felt scattered, and I worked on many projects that struggled to see me complete them. I was inefficiently active when I needed to be proficiently proactive. I impatiently looked ahead to my goals without the awareness of my intention. And to be honest, I am still learning to be powerfully present. I am slowly recognizing and understanding from an experiential viewpoint, the absolute treasure we've been given in the joy of creating.

Unfortunately, the cost of comparison has become a national crisis. However, when we value ourselves and are patient in the way that we believe our own life is meant to unwind, then we don't feel the need to compete. We take the time to rest and to indulge in sleep when it behooves us. We put our feet up, we cook a meal for ourselves before offering to do so for anyone else, and we learn to say no when we just don't have it to give. We eat mindfully and hydrate fully. We take the time

to laugh. We take frequent breaks. We move our body. We pamper ourselves. And we learn to schedule it all in.
We learn to schedule it all in, and then actually do it! For me, scheduling it all in, included not only career-related tasks, but relationship-focused ones as well as self-care rituals such as "give myself a manicure and pedicure from 3:00pm-3:45pm." In fact, I went as far as listing tasks such as phone calls to connect with friends and family.

Today, I use Office 365 to schedule, especially my business-focused meetings and goals, along with important family obligations. However, I also make use of a large white board on which I color code daily, weekly, monthly, and annual goals and projections.

It is very rare that I don't check off all my daily tasks, with what I might add, is a great deal of satisfaction. It reminds me that taking the time to plan and to organize my day, my week, and my future is a valuable focusing strategy that helps to ensure that the life I envision for myself will in fact show up!

You might say, "I don't have time to do that. I'm busy working every day, have 3 kids at home, a big house I'm trying to manage, and I'm exhausted."

Here comes the cliché: *I used to say the exact same thing!*

But it's soo true! That's why we take the time as humans to write self-help books for each other. We have a compassionate, compelling desire to share what we've learned. However, it's up to you whether or not you believe you're worth it enough to take the extra time to plan your most fabulous life!

For me, taking the time to plan, and to anticipate and feel excited about my dreams and my vision, has definitely given me a priceless ROI. More than anything, it has seen many of my dreams come to fruition, and that has brought me JOY, a feeling that for a very long time appeared to elude me.

However, I did more than invest time. I invested money. I put more and more money on the table to invest in books, seminars, trainings, master minds, mentoring, and high level business coaches.

I bought business outfits for networking which added to my "net worthing". I bought a laptop, updated my iphone, hired professional photographers, sought out sales and marketing experts, brand experts, and much more. I hesitated, less and less, as I realized the absolute value that I brought to the marketplace. More importantly, I was willing to invest in myself for my willingness to stretch, to grow, to learn and to expand, all with a passionate desire to help others. I placed currency into circulation with the utmost gratitude for what I knew it would bring back to me a millionfold.

Did you catch that last part? I PUT CURRENCY INTO CIRCULATION. Money is energy. The more we value ourselves, the more money is attracted to us, because, remember, self-worth is sexy. And it wants the best kind of relationship it can have with the most self-recognized, solid gold, always appreciated lovers that only increase in value!

It's like investing in a Trap House versus a luxury condominium in South Beach. I could crack my diamond or let it shine in all its luminescent glory!

With that being said, I want you to know that you do NOT need to protect your finances; that's fear-based and can actually scare money away. You don't need to even save money. That's like telling the Universe that you're preparing for an emergency, and so guess what? That's exactly what will show up. Spend the money, and enjoy what it can give to you and others, knowing that there will always be more. (*If you must save money, then refer to it as a "wealth" account, to be used when opportunities arise or when you'd like to have a little more fun!)

And to keep your mindset in the space of knowing there will always be more, feed your mind with uplifting music, books, videos, and movies. Surround yourself with others who are positive, grateful, compassionate, and loving. This will help to feed your spirit as well, in a way that supports the value you attribute to yourself. Settle for nothing nor no one, but the very best, as if you were hiring a contractor to secure the materials for your dream house by the sea or your yacht on the bay or your high end cabin nestled sweetly amidst a mountainous landscape.

Because part of moving beyond trauma and courageously and confidently stepping into your Most Kicka$$ Happiest, Authentic Power is knowing that you do in fact have the power to create your reality. Your most wished for wishes won't ever be denied, because contrary to what you might have once thought, there is a Higher Power to which we are ALL connected. And it always has our back. We don't need to be bought nor sold, just trust and allow our Divinity to unfold! Have faith in the new evidence as it shows up as the new loudest voice that has the ability to drown out all your past sorrows and all the doubts you may have about your tomorrows. Know that you are completely and unequivocally, completely and fully worth it!

So invest in yourself in a way that demonstrates deliciously decadent, selfish love. Practice your faith, meditate, pray, learn to respond and not react, find emotional balance, seek inner peace and equanimity amidst chaos. And also remember the second "bring the gold, that's what's happening" part of your path.

Number Two: STAND IN YOUR POWER.

This is just as important as investing in yourself when it comes to nurturing and rediscovering your *"sensational, as a birthright"*, self-worth. For you are in your Power when you stand up for who you ARE. You are in your Power when you stand up for what you believe in. You are in your Power when you refuse to compromise on your own personally identified principles. You are in your Power when you will not bend on the strength of your morals.

Not surprisingly, this power shows itself in direct correlation to your self-worth, and it exemplifies what it means to be unbreakable and unshakeable. The cool thing is that it is something you can practice. Yes, just like a homerun hitter spends hours in the batting cage and a prestigious pianist spends hours on the keys, you can practice what I mentioned above as a way to develop increasing confidence in your ability to safely speak and live your truth in the World. It naturally aligns with your Divine Design which, in turn, can't help but make you Enticingly **Happy!**

Now, I have done that myself, many times over, speaking my truth and standing up for what I believe in in a more gracious manner every time. It has allowed me to renew my faith in myself as a powerful co-creator with the ability to plant seeds into minds that may not yet be ready to grasp what I am sharing or to accept me for who I AM. This has shown itself most in relation to my view on religion. It has been a challenge to deliver my point of view to others that somehow still believe, for example, that homosexuality is "wrong, a sin, an abomination, and that it is a choice". The last aspect baffles me the most, because who in their right mind would choose something that would almost surely guarantee a life of persecution by those who deem themselves to be more righteous? And how is it a sin to express that which you were designed to be? An aberration, says Scientology. "How can that be? " I often ask others. "Is it not love that brings together two consenting adults? Where is the love and the compassion and the understanding of Divine Purpose as taught by Jesus Christ, by Buddha, by Krishna and many other prophets across all denominations?"

And so I feel obligated to share my beliefs as a way to release others from the pain of an experience not yet validated by the mainstream. However, it took me years to step into that power. I was once ashamed of who I WAS and AM, because I looked outside of me for acceptance. I looked to the masses for approval, to offer me the worth that I was not yet brave enough to unleash. And it made me feel very unhappy.

So don't worry if you're not quite ready to unveil what's already there for you. Allow yourself to remember your strength and even more so, your compassion. Be a shepherd, not a sheep. Be willing to walk to a different beat. Dare to be unique. Have the courage to lead. Speak your truth, at all times, regardless of where you might be and with whom you might be. STAND IN YOUR POWER!

Major Action Step: Begin to share an aspect about yourself that you haven't shared before, or at the very least, an aspect about yourself that still feels uncomfortable.

CHAPTER 9

Reinvent Yourself!
Create a Brand New Identity

"Yesterday I was clever, so I wanted to change the world. Today I am wise, so I am changing myself.'
— Rumi

"Life is a series of natural and spontaneous changes. Don't resist them; that only creates sorrow. Let reality be reality. Let things flow naturally forward in whatever way they like.'
— Lao Tzu

"Change in life is inevitable. We can choose to change with it, aligning ourselves with the natural flow of our destiny, or it can be forced upon us. Either way, the outcome will be the same."-Mama G

Assuming you've begun to heavily purge, and are becoming more and more comfortable with the World seeing you and hearing you just as you were designed to be, it is now time to reinvent yourself! (*Insert giddy laugh.*) Yeees! This is becoming more and more exciting, don't you think? And that's just how I believe life is meant to be; an experience of unabashed joy, heart-warming harmony, luxurious love, compelling compassion, great grace, and genuine gratitude as byproducts of passionate creation. And so let the evolution evolve as the World revolves! Think of it as a rebranding, with new eye-catching colors, new magical messaging, a new leveled up logo, and most importantly, a brand new YOU! It is the turbocharged transformed you that is preparing to take the World by storm, in a healthy viral type of way, like a jet stream that propels us forward, collapsing time and space. After all, you have been that weary traveler with multiple stop overs, a bunch of delays, on stand by for much too long. You've listened to the same song, on repeat, I repeat, on repeat, for MUCH too long.

Next stop, with a flip of the flop begins with perhaps a new theme song, one that fills your heart and gets your mojo moving and grooving; let's start there. Think of it as a talisman, something that holds magical powers to keep you energy rich! For me, it's the theme from the movie Rocky, written by Bill Conti, entitled, "Gonna Fly Now". Quite appropriate title wouldn't you say? I listen to it, and I visualize Rocky, the main character, running up the steps of the Philadelphia Museum of Art, reaching the top and then raising his fists in the air in an act of triumph.

Of course, I really sealed in this talisman by actually visiting this spot in Philadelphia while on an East Coast road trip with my kids. We ran up those same steps, and when we reached the top, we did just what Rocky did.

We jumped up, and we pumped our fists in the air. It was so much fun! If you haven't seen the movie, I would highly recommend it. For a modern day take on this movie, check out Creed. The theme song in this one is basically a rearrangement of Bill Conti's original song from the Rocky movie. Both are classic hero stories. In fact, I truly believe that that is what life is about! We all have the ability to become that hero.

And so which song do you believe would be your best "go to" song, a song that would be at the top of your most accessible playlist? Make it inspirational. Choose one that has lyrics that uplift you. A great beat or a great instrumental can get your juices going. However, if you want the "juices" to flow in a coherent, healthy pattern that helps to sustain your motivation, then keep it POSITIVE in all aspects of the song.

To be honest, a great Trap beat or a hard core heavy metal song can easily hype one up, but unless the lyrics are focusing your mind in a way that elevates your thoughts and subsequently, your mood, you may be doing yourself a great disservice by choosing this type of song. What happens in this instance is that the hype becomes like another drug, a "hit" or a "toke" that feels good in the moment, but which leaves you vibrationally lower than where you truly want to be. Choose wisely. Always choose wisely!

Moving on, let's take a look at your clothes, your outfits. It's a great time to switch up the colors, the style, to try something new. This is important, I believe, as it allows the energy of the newly transformed you to express itself in full effect! This is you stepping into your new upregulated, **Happier** Self, preparing to exhibit your innate GREATNESS to the World! It keeps you fresh like a newborn baby, YOU, rebirthed with a more readily recognized self-worth...like you went to church, but you didn't have to!

Take some time to reflect on the colors you currently feel drawn to. Look at magazines. Go online and do some window shopping. Walk down the street and see what others are wearing that might appeal to you. Then invest in that whole new wardrobe. And no matter how nice those clothes are in your closet, the jackets, the shoes, DONATE them. This is no longer you. Think about it. When a baby is born, everything is new, true? I know, I know, you may be saying to yourself, "It's not quite the same thing." Yet what if you were to take on that perspective? What if you were to completely let go, and to begin all over? What might that do for you to engage in a complete reset? Do you believe it would help you with your present mindset? Might you feel uplifted and more expansive by stepping into the frequency of clothes that align with who you are NOW?

I did just that! At one time, I wore a lot of pink and some coral. I wore pink neo adidas...classic Run DMC type sneakers with the signature 3 stripes. In fact, this is another talisman I have. When I wear these, I believe I can rap and I can freestyle like nobody's business. It's like Run DMC's in the house, and I'm resonating with their energy, like a tuning fork! At any rate, like I said, I wore a LOT of pink, and actually became known as the "pink lady". As an entrepreneur, it was in all my branding. Both my live and online presence was "pink". However, I felt a shift just before my first live event in March of 2019. I was living in Tampa, FL at the time with my then 16 year old daughter while my son attended Suffolk University in Boston, MA. My brother-in-law had transitioned 4 weeks before after a 3 $\frac{1}{2}$ year battle with cancer, and my daughter had a serious incident just 2 weeks before that. After 2 years of opportunities for what I call tremendous spiritual growth, I felt a change in the trajectory of my life. I was in a deep transformation, specifically with the way I perceived death and loss and seeming tragedy.

It was this new perspective on life, this greater awareness, that saw me throw a curve ball at my first live event. I showed up in pale blue and white with brand new neo adidas sneakers...sky blue with, of course, the signature 3 white stripes! And I felt on fire, honestly! I was so blessed to have my twin sister be a part of the event, and to have my daughter and BOTH my parents there to support me. I also had a niece and a nephew attend. Although we were all still grieving the death of my brother-in-law, there was a lightness in the room. It felt like the sky was opening up to receive me, as if to say, you passed. You have now earned a respite. You may now prepare to fly, to fly, just like the monarch butterflies born in late Summer, with the grit and the perseverance, and the grace to go out and enjoy what life has to offer. *(Interestingly enough, my deceased partner has often showed up as a monarch butterfly. ☺)*

Fast forward 2 months, I received a strong inclination to move. This was supported by a visit to South Beach in late April of 2019. A month later, I met with a realtor, put the house up for sale, and arrived in South Beach on July 2, 2019, just in time for fireworks on the beach and the bay! It was as if I had just gained my independence from the former version of who I had been, and was being celebrated for the courage to make massive change once again!

Remember from chapter 6, that I had completed a MAJOR purge! I had welcomed new clothes, a new home, a new city, a

new car, new branding, and a new outlook on life! I had even
shaved my head! And so once again, with which colors are you
currently resonating? What styles are calling you? Is it time
to step up your "A" game, to invest in some high quality outfits,
so that you can attract high quality people and opportunities?
I believe, "YES!" because YOU are worth it!

Now, what about your car.? Oh, yes, the car, too! I want to
remind you that everything carries an energy signature, and
that car is attached to your former, outdated energy
signature, the one with the version of you that was not yet
ready to step into your <u>Authentic Power</u>, the one that was run
down and depressingly decrepit. So let's have at it! How does
it feel to drive your car? Is it perhaps time to trade it in or to
buy a new one? Is it time for an update, to enjoy the
technology of blue tooth and an ability to sense when objects
are too close? Might you consider a different make or model
this time around? How about the color? Would you like a
sporty car, a more practical car, perhaps a sun roof? It's all
yours to choose! You decide! After all, it's your life, and it's
your JOY ride!

Okay, let's keep going! How's the J.O.B. or the career looking?
Is money coming in drips and drabs, and I emphasize the
"drabs"? Do you feel like you want to do more to help create
the type of lifestyle you desire?

Are you jumping out of bed, excited about the day, no matter
what day it is, or are you dreading Monday and desperately
waiting on Friday? How about your branding? Does it feel right
for you? Do you wish you had more clarity, more laser sharp
focus about exactly what it is you believe you are meant to do?

Be honest!

My guess is that regardless of where you are on your path, there is always room for growth, especially if you're reading this book!

Guess what, though! You do NOT have to figure it out today! Patience, self-reflection, and taking the time to breathe in greater awareness IS action. It's this type of action that keeps you from grinding, pushing through, and feeling fatally frazzled!! Better to skip the frazzle, and instead properly prepare for a little razzle dazzle after a solid phase of rejuvenation and renewal. The key, however, is to make that decisive move when you know you are ready. If you seem to be languishing in elongated, drawn out spa days, I suggest you put the book down, leave poolside, put on your theme song, and start taking that next action step!

To conclude, we all have greatness within us! And when we learn to access this greatness, it naturally elevates our mood, bringing us true **Happiness**. I believe this goes without question. However, not everyone is brave enough to let go, and to make the kind of change that is necessary to access this greatness. Transformation is an ongoing life process. Change is inevitable. Creating your own course of change is a preferable and more graceful way to transform your life. But again, as I just mentioned, change is inevitable, just like the clouds come and go in the sky, so do moments in our lives. Change, we must. Any resistance to the natural order of things will only result in a forced, dramatic, tumultuous, tumbling down wakeup call. And so let this book be your guide, your proactive toolbox with the DIY, get it done NOW, while there is still some air in the tires and some charge in the battery. Even if you opt for the tow truck, like I did at one time, there is always the opportunity to make a different choice. ☺

Major Action Step: Change at least one aspect of your life that you are committed to changing RIGHT NOW, TODAY.

CHAPTER 10

Start Being You!
Authenticity as an Earmark to a Phenomenal Life

"Confidence is created by the small things you do every day that allow you to build trust in yourself."
-Mel Robbins

"Do one thing every day that scares you."
-Eleanor Roosevelt

"Be who you are, always, regardless of where you are and who you're with." -Mama G

Wow! I can sense you lighting up! You ARE in fact, facilitating your own change! You are taking "Double D, 4G, LED" charge of your own **happiness!** This is magnificently marvelous! You're on all pistons, well out of the breakdown lane, and traveling at a pretty decent velocity on the free way of life! It's like the top is popped, the sun is shining brightly and you can feel an exhilarating wind waking up all of your senses! You feel fearless, courageous, bodacious, and are ready to get outrageous, whatever it takes, to let the World know you have, in fact, arrived! You have survived, and now it's time to thrive! So why stop now! Keep cruising, keep perusing all the endless possibilities! You are grand, and your life can be grand!

This is the point on your journey where you are presented with countless choices, all wondrous! You have earned the keys to unlock your limitless power! Use them to speak your truth with grace and ease every opportunity you have. In fact, create those opportunities. Share your story! Share your triumph! Know that you belong just as you are, that you are perfect in your design, that you absolutely have something extremely and supremely powerful to contribute to others and to the planet!

Continue to grow. Step out of your comfort zone every single day, multiple times a day, if you feel so inclined! Stretch your mind, reach for the stars, and know that there is always more! More, more, more, always!

Do those LIVE videos, wear that sassy outfit, pull out that 2-piece bathing suit. Jump on a jet ski, take a cruise to the Bahamas, try surfing, go skinny dipping, climb a mountain, tour the country in an RV! Order wine, coffee, AND tiramisu! Attend an open mic, learn a new language, test drive a Ferrari. Express more and more of your unconditional love! Hug your clients! Pet dogs, caress cats, talk to strangers, talk to your plants!

Step on stage, and bring your gifts to the World for all to see. Be visible. Be seen. Shine in all your glory, exuding the most flavorful, fall in love **Kicka$$ Happyness** you can!

Be YOU! Be Real. Be Transparent. Be Authentic. Be Great!

And most importantly...
Be Happy!!!

APPENDIX A
(GOLDEN MILK RECIPE)

Golden Milk Recipe

Perfect for an evening drink just before bed; here's Dr. Weil's recipe for Golden Milk:

- Heat 2 cups light, unsweetened coconut milk (or almond or soymilk)
- Add 1/2 tablespoon peeled, grated fresh ginger
- Add 1 tablespoon peeled, grated fresh turmeric
- Add 3-4 black peppercorns

Heat all ingredients in a saucepan

- Stir well
- Bring to a simmer and simmer covered for 10 minutes.
- Strain and sweeten to taste (if desired).

APPENDIX B
(ALTERNATIVE HEALING MODALITES)

As humans, we desperately want to fit in, to feel loved, to be accepted. Below is a partial list of alternative modalities that have been known to produce dramatic results for those who wish to expedite their own personal transformation by addressing the mind, body, spirit connection.

1. Access Bars
2. Acupuncture
4. Aromatherapy
5. ASMR Therapy (Autonomous Sensory Meridian Response)
6. Astrology
7. Bemer Therapy
8. Chiropractic Care
9. Cold Laser Therapy
10. Cranial-structure therapy
11. Crystal Therapy
12. Cupping
13. EMDR Therapy (Eye Movement Desensitization and Reprocessing)
14. Essential Oils
15. Flower Essences
16. Foot Baths
17. Hypnosis
18. Kundalini Yoga (Vril Power)
19. Scalar Light Therapy
20. Meditation
21. Mindfulness
22. MPS (Dolphin) Therapy
23. Past Life Regression
24. Polarity Massage
25. Prayer
26. Reiki

27.   Reconnective Healing
28.   Reflexology
29.   Shamanic Healing
30.   Sonic Healing
31.   Sound Healing
32.   Structural Energetic Therapy (SET)
33.   Tai Chi
34.   Therapeutic Massage
35.   Yoga

*FYI...I've done ALL of these and MORE!

APPENDIX C
(POWER OF THOUGHT RESOURCES)

Books...

Hung by the Tongue by Martin Francis
As a Man Thinketh by James Allen
Think and Grow Rich by Napoleon Hill
Psycho-Cybernetics by Maxwell Maltz
Ask and You Shall Receive by Maria F. La Riva (*e-book)
The Science of Mind by Ernest Holmes
The Science of Belief by Bruce Lipton
The Master Key System by Charles F. Haanel
The Secret by Rhonda Byrne (and company)
Law of Attraction by Esther and Jerry Hicks
The Science of Success by William Wattles
Becoming Supernatural by Joe Dispenza
The Placebo Effect by Joe Dispenza
Thoughts are Things by Bob Proctor
The Divine Matrix by Gregg Braden
The Isaiah Effect by Gregg Braden
The Power of Positive Thinking by Dr. Norman Vincent Peale

YouTube...

https://www.youtube.com/user/YouAreCreators/videos
https://www.youtube.com/channel/UCxl847Lx10jCdq1wkLPp3v
g/videos

https://www.youtube.com/user/BobProctorTV/videos

Meet the Author

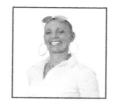

Anne Hayes (aka Mama G), THE EMPOWERMENT QUEEN, is a speaker, author, poet, rapper, reiki master/trainer and a spiritual reconnection specialist. She and her team provide transformational programs that empower individuals to achieve breakthrough results in both life and business.

Anne has over 30 years of experience working with teens and youth as a teacher in both the public and the private sectors, as well as a community outreach worker in urban neighborhoods. Her mission is to create a global community of joyful and fulfilled teens who support each other in making the World a better place.

She currently resides in Miami Beach, FL, U.S.A. with her teenage daughter. She loves to write, swim, spend time with family and friends, and enjoys a daily meditation practice with yoga.

She is also the author of <u>Teenage Grace/La Gracia del Joven</u>, a compilation of meditations for especially the Teenage Spirit.

Furthermore, she is a leader and an advocate for the LGBTQ Community.

To learn more about Anne Hayes (AKA Mama G), go to <u>https://annehayes360.com/</u>.

WITH MUCH LOVE,

ANNE HAYES/MAMA G ☺

Made in the USA
Columbia, SC
09 March 2020

88654102R00065